COLOR MEDICINE

CHARLES KLOTSCHE

The secrets of
color/vibrational healing

COLOR MEDICINE

The Secrets of
Color/Vibrational Healing

Charles Klotsche

COLOR MEDICINE
The Secrets of Color/Vibrational Healing

© Copyright by Charles Klotsche

Published by
Light Technology Publishing
P.O. Box 1526, Sedona, AZ 86336, U.S.A.
ISBN 0-929385-27-6

Cover photograph courtesy of Dr. Bara H. Fischer

Printed by Mission Possible Commercial Printing
in Sedona, Arizona, U.S.A.

Dedication

We live in an age where the material has become separated from the spiritual. Everything we seemingly have is physical, mechanical, mortal, lineal and finite. We tend to be individuals at the expense of everything else. In reality, we are not absolute entities, but are linked by a state of energy where no division between human beings, atoms and molecules is discernible.

A new process is emerging, one that includes the whole being. This process is a manifestation of the material, psychological and spiritual entity, a recognizable essential in the effective process of healing the human body.

Color Medicine is dedicated to my two daughters, Lyna and Kelly, who, like a multitude of others, are becoming one with the unraveling mysteries of life and the perceivable and discoverable laws of the universe.

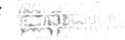

Acknowledgments

Charles Klotsche acknowledges Dr. Dinshah P. Ghadiali, the East Indian physician, and his three-volume series entitled *Spectro-Chrome-Metry Encyclopaedia* (copyright 1933, 1934) for his pioneering research in the field of color medicine, or vibrational healing. Many of Dinshah's ideas and methods were an impetus to, and are incorporated into, *Color Medicine.*

To Dr. Bara Fischer whose invaluable research and input made this manuscript a reality, a special thanks.

Thanks also to Margaret Pinyan for her editorial assistance and indefatigable support for excellence in this book.

A Note from the Author

When I became interested in studying the physical healing sciences I was initially inspired to look for alternative healing methods in a specific attempt to understand contemporary disease as it relates to the physical and energy bodies. Subsequently I explored the metaphysical aspects, especially those related to the subtle-energy fields surrounding the body and those specifically associated with holistic healing.

With time, I became interested in the characteristics of how subtle energy vibrations permeated human beings, and how alternative healing methods utilized these vibratory patterns of the universe. I experienced chiropractors, for instance, rechannel this life-supporting energy to the needed areas of the body merely by adjusting the spine. I witnessed acupuncturists recirculate this energy through virtually unseen meridian systems that connected this subatomic energy with atomic organs located deep within the human body. I met healers who, utilizing only their hands, moved around certain energies similar to those found in the higher octaves of the electromagnetic scale where they actually increased or decreased the vibrational activity in the body. These activities all had one common thread — the utilization of the subtle energy vibrations, in effect similar to those found in the visible spectrum — the 49th octave — of the universe's electromagnetic scale, manifesting in light that we can see.

In the process of my investigations, I discovered an interesting breakthrough, as old as recorded medicine itself, that can recirculate blocked energy in the physical realm through a higher energy process used as vibrational healing or color medicine. This is a technique that dates back to at least 500 B.C. and was utilized by Pythagoras and others. With additional time and research, much of which dealt with Eastern teachings, I found this concept to be on the cutting edge of both mystical and spiritual beliefs as well as completely in harmony with state-of-the-art sophisticated and contemporary techniques utilized for alternative healing. As I now perceive it, color medicine makes a truly multidimensional contribution to the advancement and betterment of human life. With time and patience I have ascertained that this is an incredibly powerful method for strengthening the human immune system in a safe and cost-effective manner. Combining aura-attuned chromatherapy with harmonious sounds, tissue salts and hydrochroma-therapy further reinforces this powerful therapy, resulting in The 49th Vibrational Technique.

I came to realize that few individuals are totally satisfied with the contemporary methods used in the healing process. In my travels I began to sense a degree of hopelessness prevailing in society at large, especially as it related to those in the middle or advanced stages of the aging process. I had a feeling that, metaphorically, many were running on six instead of eight cylinders, without the access or ability to tune themselves up effectively.

I often thought humanity was denied or being cut off from the instruction or repair manuals for dealing with their own bodies because of the way contemporary medicine has been practiced. I wondered whether anyone would or could provide the necessary repairs to this system at the present critical point in time. It is for this reason that The 49th Vibrational Technique came into being, as I had to be assured of the existence of a satisfactory support system to the self-healing process, at least for nondegenerative types of diseases. I have attempted in the pages that follow to encapsulate an encyclopedia of the knowledge I have obtained on color medicine in a condensed and nonanecdotal form. Additional volumes can and will be written, stressing supportive empirical evidence collected and documented by positive results achieved through The 49th Vibrational Technique and other contributing variations of color medicine and natural healing.

Since my initial probing into the alternative or holistic healing process, many of my views have changed — for the better. Many of the same doors will be open to you as you progress through the realms of in-depth understanding of how and under what conditions the human body can best function.

Charles Klotsche, Founder/President
The 49th Vibration, Inc.

Table Of Contents

CHAPTER 3

COLOR HARMONICS:
The Twelve Healing Colors and Their Use

COLOR PRACTICE:
Materials and Practical Techniques for Applying Color Medicine

C H A P T E R   5

COLOR SCHEDULE APPLICATION:
Determining the Appropriate Color(s) for Relieving/Healing the 123 Major Illnesses

APPENDIX

LIST OF DIAGRAMS

LIST OF TABLES

Foreword

Does Color Medicine Really Heal?

A Book on Esoteric Physics

This book and its esoteric, yet science-related, material on color medicine and other related subjects will change your entire perception of how the healing process works. It brings forward a new, more realistic understanding of healing. By esoteric we mean energies that individuals can learn to sense or visualize and ultimately use for purposes of healing even though present-day science has no instruments to measure or comprehend them. Fortunately, in this endeavor old taboos no longer hinder the search for solutions in the age of enlightenment.

Healing Beyond Today's Accepted Understanding

Some think chromatherapy is a combination of mystical and spiritual knowledge. Conceivably it is, although it can be explained scientifically in terms of the wavelengths and vibrations described in any college-level physics textbook. However, becoming one with the so-called mysteries of life and the laws of the universe means one must reorient one's systems of beliefs and values. After all, we have equal access to levels of higher consciousness and other sophisticated methods of dealing with ourselves and the diseases found within our bodies.

The human body is a cellular vehicle operating on a modular level, according to contemporary medical science. This branch of science historically has had a tendency to ignore the fact that the body is comprised of a network of higher and lower energy fields – some measurable, some not, at least by conventional means.

These interrelating systems of subtle forces recharge or rechannel energy into diseased areas where it is blocked or deficient, for disease is nothing more than a restriction of energy flows. As we know, energy or vibrations flow along the path of least resistance, and, through the extra energy associated with the use of vibrational healing, the appropriate energies seek out the needed areas, freeing blocked energy where it is most required. The interaction between the dense physical energy of the body and the subtle energy, which controls many of the body functions or activities, is the key to understanding the relationship between energy and matter.

The Healing Base of The 49th Vibrational Technique, or Reinforcing Color Medicine

Applying the appropriate color wavelengths or vibrations to the human body is transforming the present practice of contemporary medicine beyond recognition. This practice will accelerate geometrically as man learns that disease, at least in its nondegenerate form, is nothing but a temporary blockage or disturbance of the vital life force in the body.

The 49th octave, here called _49th vibrational range_ or _49th vibration_, is scientifically referred to as a narrow band in the cosmic electromagnetic energy spectrum, known to mankind as the visible color spectrum. It is composed of reds, greens and blues and their combined derivatives, producing the perceivable colors that fall between the ultraviolet and the infrared ranges of energy or vibrations. These visual colors, with their unique wavelengths and oscillations – when combined with a light source — provide the necessary healing energy the body requires when selectively applied to the impaired organs or life systems.

The 49th Vibrational Technique utilizes the twelve most powerful of these visible colors for healing. Each of its twelve selected colors vibrates at hundreds of trillions of times per second, interfacing with the blocked or distorted energy in the physical body through a unique oscillation process. The 49th Vibrational Technique assigns a predetermined frequency to each color selected from the visible spectrum whose particular vibrations either raise, lower or neutralize energy levels as necessary in specific parts of the body to aid the self-healing or holistic health process. What makes this method so unique and powerful?

Color medicine is not governed by laws of the physical plane alone — at least as third-dimensional man relates to them. It is not definable in lineal, rational terminology, nor does it contain the restrictions or finite boundaries set up by the preconceived, often distorted assortment of human beliefs. When one assumes a multidimensional attitude toward healing that is open for events beyond the laws of the physical plane, then much of the sophisticated technology developed by those who are attached mainly to the physical world and its inherent trappings becomes obsolete.

Our concept is premised on the idea that on the surface of the skin the physical and etheric (energy) bodies interface through the color vibrations found and utilized by The 49th Vibrational Technique. Light affects both the physical and etheric bodies. Our twelve vibrating colors generate electrical impulses and magnetic currents or fields of energy that are prime activators of the biochemical and hormonal process in the human body, the stimulants or sedatives necessary to balance the entire system and its organs.

As pure white light enters the body, it refracts similar to the way light refracts and disperses into many colors when it passes through a prism. The various color shades that travel through the body not only have unique color vibrations, but they also have chemical equivalents; reds being stimulating (hydrogen) and blues being soothing (oxygen). Each color has its own wavelength, which can be attuned to the other colors (or vibrations) to alter a function or balance the system. It is analogous to the way musical notes are tuned to each other to achieve harmony. By inserting the necessary colors (vibrations) into the body's energy system, the vital life force again flows naturally.

Unlike many other chromatherapy systems, The 49th Vibrational Technique uses a proven scientific color healing system that it reinforces with aura harmonics: attuned color-sounds, related tissue salts, supportive hydrochromatherapy and assigned astrological color rays. These color harmonics help the healing colored lights to readjust and sustain the perfect vibrancy of each person between therapy sessions. This reinforcement by aura harmonics makes The 49th Vibration Technique particularly powerful.

Energy/Matter — Dual Expressions of an Identical Substance

The Western world appears to be trapped in the mechanistic approaches — ignoring the energy nature of man, where disease can be healed by energy or color vibrations. Modern science views the healing process as a kind of Newtonian concept based upon formulas of mechanistic or functional, reactional behavior derived from the visually observable processes of the material world. The process is based upon acceleration and gravity, studied by Newton, who structured these ideas into a variety of mathematical laws pertaining to physical action and reaction.

The Newtonian concept of calculus gave impetus to the scientific community to structure the tools that more accurately measured and defined the observable universe, providing in the process unthought-of ideas and inventions — many of which contributed to the industrial revolution, individual specialization of employment, and the general mechanization of Western society.

By further refining this mechanistic concept of the identifiable, the scientific community formulated the basis for determining how most of the present-day mechanical systems would or should operate.

Conceptually, Newtonian ideas helped us to understand solid matter — that is, moving objects found in the earth's gravitational field — but his concepts are incapable of dealing with electricity and magnetism and their interactions with living systems and the universe at large.

Newtonian concepts — limited to the observable — have also been applied by contemporary medicine, which premises its concept on the idea that the total picture becomes predictable by understanding and regulating the various material parts. That is, when a part of the body malfunctions, it is removed or replaced, the same way we handle machinery. Alternatively, it is treated with chemical ingredients which often cause negative side effects. Simply stated, contemporary medicine looks at the symptoms and influences or suppresses them, but does not involve itself with the *real* source: diseased life energy.

Einstein, on the other hand, through his renowned equation, $E = mc^2$, determined that energy and matter are dual expressions of an identical universal substance. This means that there are finer energy sources at work in living systems besides the readily observable and mechanical interactions — thus going beyond the Newtonian approach.

Color medicine combines both approaches and deals in the widest framework of all, the body's essential spiritual and physical life energy. Yet it is surprisingly easy to explain in the simplest of frameworks, as we will show you with The 49th Vibrational Technique.

Spiritual and Materialistic Concepts of Energy Medicine

Western thought appears to be influenced by Egypt, a stronghold of culture, religion and art for an incredible period of 3000 years. The East looked to India, which was a leader in philosophy, culture and art — a society as ancient as Egypt. However, they took different or diametrically opposed approaches (from BioElectric Evaluation Mediation [B.E.E.M.] research).

Egyptians visualized the way to wholeness through discipline of the mind; India through discipline of the body. Since body and mind form a unity, imbalances in both approaches were bound to surface with time.

The Egyptian philosophy resulted in a rigidity of mind, with its material concerns and solutions as preeminent requirements established by the rational mind. India, on the other hand, developed yoga to discipline the body, disregarding its needs and desires for the comforts found in the material world. Spiritual (that is, energetic) concerns and solutions played a role first in India, unfortunately neglecting the body in the process. However, the Indian vastness of unrestricted thought allowed them to see the illusion called matter — a fact only Einstein could prove to a materialistic/mechanized, Newton-bound world of the West through his mathematical energy formula $E = mc^2$.

According to Einstein, energy and matter are interchangeable and interconvertible. We see this through the process of converting matter into energy, and energy back into matter. If we look to the matter (mass) side of $E = mc^2$, we can visualize the tremendous amount of potential energy condensed in a particle of matter. We know that matter, for instance, can be converted into energy as demonstrated by the atomic bomb, where a small amount of matter (uranium) releases enough energy to destroy a city.

By uniting the Egyptian and East Indian approaches (combining matter and energy) and applying them properly, as in The 49th Vibrational Technique, the energies of the visible light spectrum release tremendous healing powers in the physical body.

Mass or matter (m) accelerated by the square of the speed of light (c^2) becomes dematerialized energy (E), meaning that the basis of all material substance in nature is energy. Only with the Einstein formula, satisfying the Egyptian analytic mind, could the West finally break away from the Egyptian analysis, materialism and restriction of the mind — finally creating a departure from seeking rapid solutions through symptom analysis. Only through hunger and suffering could India — lost alive in the vastness of the spiritual realm — become aware of a vibrational essence for comforting the body: color medicine.

Thus, Einstein's formula $E = mc^2$ expanded the consciousness of the West toward seeing the oneness of all creation beyond duality — and proved that the application of Eastern light therapy (c) on the body (m) would effectively work (E).

However, color medicine, or vibrational therapy, like all healing arts, must function in relationship to a particular frame of reference, whether physical, psychological or spiritual, or (as in the case of The 49th Vibrational Technique) a combination of the three. Energy, being the spiritual body of man, equals the physical (m) times light (c^2).

How Vibratory Rates Determine Density and Form

The Einstein approach deals with the human body not as an assemblage of parts or chemicals but as a total, complete system operating in harmony with the electromagnetic/energy system of the universe, similar to the way in which the Eastern philosophy of medicine understands the physical/energy connection.

The key to understanding vibrational healing, or color medicine, lies not in the Newtonian mechanistic approach — physically repairing or removing cellular material — but in rerouting energy fields that form complicated relationships with other fields such as those surrounding the physical/cellular substance and others relating to more nonphysical energies. These energies flow through the body, continually materializing and then reverting back to energy.

For instance, we know that the vibratory rate of a substance determines its density or its form as matter. Slow-vibrating substance is often referred to as physical matter — whereas the subatomic (that which vibrates at or above the speed of light) is subtle (subatomic) matter, or pure light energy.

All these specific arrays of vibrations are either harmonizing, neutralizing or distorting each other — or, in terms of healing, are beneficial or detrimental to the human body. The vibratory rates inherent to The 49th Vibrational Technique are such that they balance any diseased energy pattern found in the body. For in every organ there is an energetic level at which the organ best functions. Any departure from that vibratory rate results in pathology, whereas restoring the appropriate energy levels to the physical organs results in a healed body.

How Color Vibrations Function as an Electrical Transformer

The 49th Vibrational Technique's energy-reallocation system functions much like the standard electrical transformer, shifting and redirecting the electromagnetic energies that pass through the body. The violet end of the spectrum relieves energy overloads, the red end generally stimulates the nonfunctioning or underfunctioning parts of the system, and the green center provides a neutral or stabilizing effect. The 49th Vibrational Technique provides the complete or composite polarity process needed to enhance the body's energy. As in electromagnetic fields, positive, neutral and negative are also characteristic of the twelve colors we utilize.

Even some branches of contemporary medicine recognize that disease in a nondegenerative form is simply a blockage of vital energy in the organs, atoms, tissues or body systems. Only the methods and results of treatment differ from color medicine. To facilitate healing, The 49th Vibrational Technique works with the appropriate vibratory rates needed by the different body areas. For example, the healthy heart vibrates differently from the healthy spleen and consequently needs a different vibratory rate when out of balance. Therefore, The 49th Vibrational Technique systematically matches twelve different sources of vibrations in the visible color spectrum with the needs of major energy centers or energy pathways in the human body. This healing system can thus effectively eliminate the source of most nondegenerative and some degenerative diseases or energy blockages in the human body without mutilation (surgery) or drugs if applied in time.

Even though the list of diseases that have been reversed through color medicine is quite comprehensive today, not all have been curable without resort to radical medical means. Unfortunately, some of the degenerative diseases may be beyond reversibility through color medicine.

When we recognize the vibratory patterns in the universe — that is, the energy ranges or fields found on the cosmic electromagnetic scale — we will then be able to open the doors to the tremendous healing powers found in the subtle-energy octaves of the cosmos. The visible light spectrum, with its beneficial frequencies for the human body, provides a disease-preventing tool for healing. Color medicine is truly the medicine of the future.

Holistic Healing — Simply Balancing Polarities

Current science tends to lead to ever greater complexity, causing a feeling of disempowerment in the individual. We seem to be creating a society where no one is supposed to claim authority in any field other than his own approved specialty. This is particularly alarming when current mechanistic medical practice still claims exclusive authority over the vital functions affecting life and death. However, some practitioners within the medical community are receiving increasing attention for their holistic approach to health, which has been carried on by naturopathic physicians during the dominance of allopathy. Hopefully, this demonstrates that a change is on the way that will simplify the issue of health and further support individual self-empowerment, as does The 49th Vibrational Technique. This technique is structured for the individual to use. It is simple and practical in nature, providing everyone with cost-effective solutions or alternatives to healing the human body — thus enabling individuals to assume sovereignty over their own health destiny.

Color Medicine unequivocally demonstrates to the reader how to improve or reverse the adverse or deficient energy in the body through the use of appropriate, reinforcing or counteracting colors or vibrations. When the deficient energy is balanced with the proper polarity (south/north, negative/positive, female/male, blues/reds), The 49th Vibrational Technique will unleash the counteractive energies or vibrations necessary for solving the mystery of more than 100 of the most common diseases known to mankind (see Chapter 5). The 49th Vibrational Technique permits the life energy to again flow unobstructed, healing most, if not all, nondegenerative diseases in the process, and often improving even degenerative ailments.

Utilizing the Ancient-New Technique

Color medicine is as old as recorded medicine itself, although it has been virtually dormant during the last several centuries in the West. Another branch of vibrational healing, sound therapy, is successfully pursued through subliminal tapes on the market, but it can be even more effective when used with attuned color frequencies. Like Cinderella, holistic healing and color medicine are finally making it to the ball, this time without the negation of their credibility and with fewer legal obstacles from the bastions of orthodox medicine. *Color Medicine* covers the most important aspects of vibrational medicine and color/music therapy associated with the healing process. With this publication you can master the necessary techniques of healing through color and sound. Here, in one volume, is a composite healing system for the Golden Age.

This book is laid out in such a fashion that it permits you to progress logically through all the necessary healing steps. First are the essential physics/esoteric concepts that underlie the color-therapy process. Next come the application of the twelve colors and sound vibrations and the explanation of how they effectively balance one's energy levels. Following that is the complete information necessary for the reader to acquire most cost-effectively the necessary equipment (the light source and color filters). A full explanation about the conditions under which color medicine best functions is also provided. A special section is devoted to the use of sound as a supplement to the healing process. Finally, a complete guide is provided for the 123 most common dis-eases and how health can be improved by the various applications of our 12 vibrating colors. Each "disease," in alphabetical order, is correlated to a specific color(s) or series of vibrations for improvement. You will find a Quick-Reference Checklist for color application at the end of the book.

This comprehensive work was done to enable its readers to progress through the color- and sound-therapy process, from the overview or conceptual phase all the way through details of practical application, offering an opportunity for simple self-healing. *Color Medicine* presents the entire color and sound vibrational picture, showing you the extraordinary opportunities available in vibrational therapy. Reprogram yourself with the following pages and learn of the healing potentials of color and sound therapy.

1

Color Physics

The Scientific Explanation
of Color Medicine, or
Vibrational Therapy

The 49th Vibrational Technique beneficially influences man simultaneously on the different levels of his existence: the physical, psychological and spiritual planes – all connected by the mind for an integrated understanding. Since these levels interact with each other but are perceivable as different energy worlds, we will investigate the functions and effects of vibrations on each level separately for a better comprehension of the whole.

The Newtonian Theory of Color

Most of today's fundamental understanding of color can be attributed to Isaac Newton in the 17th century. Prior to Newton's work, color was thought to be an attribute inherent to every object and contained within the object itself. Newton disproved this idea and replaced it with the notion that light falling upon the object was the way it received color. Light, of course, is the true source of color — color understood in the wave aspect of light.

The concept that colors are contained in white light is demonstrated through the use of a glass prism. By shining a beam of light through a prism, light is dispersed into the spectrum of the seven colors: red, orange, yellow, blue, green, indigo and violet (see Diagram 1-1).

We observe that when light passes into a prism the rays are bent, or refracted (Diagram 1-1), which is also true for light when traveling into any other medium. For instance, if one looks at an object in a lake from above the surface of the water and attempts to reach for that object, one will probably miss it on the first attempt, because the light refracted from the water's surface visually displaces the object from its actual location.

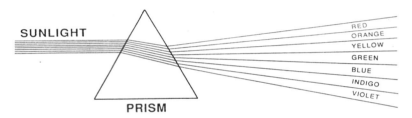

Diagram 1-1. Refraction (bending) and dispersion (scattering). When leaving a prism, light is dispersed. This refraction and dispersion separates white light into its component color rays.

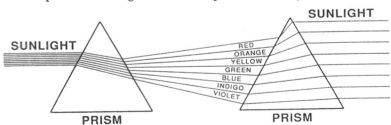

Diagram 1-2. Newton's experiment. Newton took the experiment of Diagram 1-1 further when he put a second prism in the path of the projected light after it had been diffused from the first prism. When the spectrum of the rainbow passed through the second prism, the light turned pure white again.

Experiments with two prisms show that, depending on the angle of light and the placement of the prisms, the white light from the second prism may also appear when light passes directly through that prism. Is there a possibility that the white rays, coming out of the second prism, overlay the colored rays that have passed through both prisms and make them invisible? Additional research may prove or disprove this.

Newton concluded from his experiment that there could be no further basic colors available in the universe, because the seven rainbow colors returned to their original pure-white state. Through his experiment, Newton concluded that the source of all color is white light.

Goethe's Color Theory: Boundaries Make the Colors

A departure from Newton's theory that refraction and dispersion create colors can be found in Goethe's color theory recorded prior to 1810. This theory is still not totally accepted, even though it is successfully applied in modern achromatic telescopes. By studying prisms with color plates, Goethe recognized that the boundaries of light and darkness are necessary to create colors.

Colors arise, according to Goethe, immediately after light enters a prism, a fact he proved with water prisms. He found that neither refraction nor dispersion can be the *cause* of the prismatic colors; it is instead the interaction of light and darkness through the edges of the prism. In other words, refraction itself creates no colors.

Although Goethe's and Newton's color theories differ in many ways, they both agree that rays of white light contain seven different colors — which are the healing wavelengths that we use in color medicine.

The Physics of Light and Color

It is commonly understood that the seven rainbow colors are the result of the disintegration of white light into its components, the colors. We then can say that the dispersion of light seen in the various colors relates directly to the length of the light waves themselves. The waves of the seven rainbow colors vary in length, which is the distance from the crest of one wave through its trough to the crest of the following wave. Each color has its own unique wavelength.

In a prism, the longer waves are refracted less than the shorter waves (bent least). Since red has the longest wavelength in the visible color spectrum, the red wave is the least refracted color wave when sent through a glass prism (Diagram 1-1), followed by orange, yellow, green, blue, and indigo, in that order. At the other end of the spectrum, violet light has a wavelength that is the most refracted (bent most) of the color waves.

As we look at the seven basic colors emerging from a prism, there is a reliable sequential order to the arrangement of the spectral colors. Each color relates to a particular wavelength, or vibration, on the visible spectrum. Put differently, a particular vibration (wavelength) is inherent in each spectral color. These color vibrations, which can also be regarded as energies, can produce healing effects when the appropriate wavelengths (colors) are used. Many colors, however, are a mixture of several color frequencies. Although these are used in other color healing systems, they are not as effective as the distinct frequency colors, prismatic colors, that we use. Since the shades of one color vary somewhat in terms of their wavelengths, it is important to get the precisely correct, aura-attuned shades for healing. The exact frequency cannot be determined by the eye.

In physics, light or color rays are characterized by their specific wavelength (that is, measurement in space) and frequency (measurement in time). As the rays accelerate (raise their speed, or frequency), their wavelengths are shortened.

We can see from Diagram 1-3 that the entire visible light band (known as the 49th octave, or 49th vibration) falls within a quite minuscule range among the vast array of wavelengths in the universe. Past one end of this visible range, where its shortest wavelengths are found, are the ultraviolet waves; at the other end, containing its longest waves, are found the infrareds and radio waves. Of course, waves extend farther out on both ends of the spectrum, but are not considered here for the purposes of color medicine.

Waves are a function of vibration consisting of wavelength and oscillation rate as parameters of physics. For example, in The 49th Vibrational Technique, red has the longest wavelength and the lowest

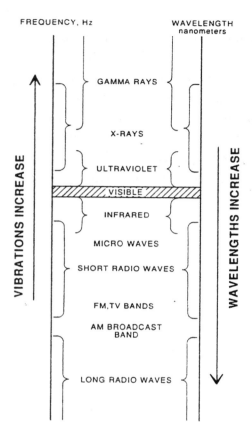

Diagram 1-3. The electromagnetic spectrum, vibrations of the universe. The visible spectrum, marked with diagonal lines, has been termed the 49th vibrational range. Radio waves, at the bottom of this scale, are slower/longer than gamma rays at the top, which are faster/shorter. The audio spectrum is located around the 9th vibrational range (4th–15th octave).

vibratory rate of the visible range, oscillating 397 trillion times per second. Violet, the color with the shortest wavelength and the highest vibratory rate, oscillates 665 trillion times per second. Green, in the middle of the spectrum, vibrates at 531 trillion times per second (Diagram 1-4). These findings are based on the theory that light moves in waves. However, there is another point of view.

The Dual Nature of Light: Wave or Particle?

Much has been said about the way in which light moves. Some schools supported the wave theory; others preferred the particle theory. Finally, Louis de Broglie received the Nobel Prize in 1929 for uniting the two theories. His work makes clear that the opposing characteristics of energy as "immaterial" waves and "substantial" particles are united to form light. To understand how these two states of light functions could work together, let us imagine that light moves in spirals. White light, containing all color frequencies, would be composed of spirals of different sizes for each color wave. Where the spirals' paths meet, a

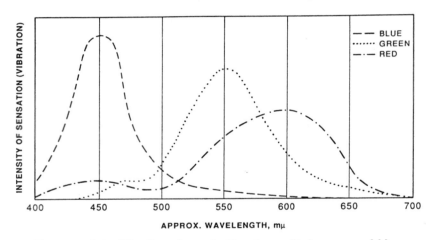

Diagram 1-4. **Wavelengths and vibrations.** Red, green and blue, three of the colors used in The 49th Vibrational Technique.

compact charge situation would occur, and particles (i.e., photons, still a nonmaterial form of energy) would be created. These photons may even move along the spiral and disappear again "outside" of it. By this "spiral path theory" (B.E.E.M. research) a laser could be understood as a ray one coil wide made of several intertwined spirals to create a single color.

Thus light has wave properties (spirals) as well as particle properties (meeting point of two or more spirals), a charge situation. But the proof for either of these properties of light necessitates a different experimental approach. For instance, let us say that one has a plastic bag filled with marbles and water (suggested by B.E.E.M.). To prove that the bag contains marbles (particles), we would bang it on a hard surface to listen for the sound of colliding marbles – the equivalent of proving the particle theory of light. To prove that the bag contains water (waves), we would press it repeatedly, noting that it moved like a waterbed – similar to proving the wave theory of light.

Only by combining the two concepts can we see the entire picture. The bag contains both marbles and water – that is, light is made up of both particles and waves. To more easily comprehend the properties of light and color, we will now consider the wave characteristic of light.

How Objects Receive Color – Absorption and Reflection

Although color is inherent in any vibration, it is interesting to note that it is our eyes that translate some of the energy waves of objects and forces of life into perceivable forms that appear to us in a variety of colors. As the various wavelengths of white light affect our vision, we then must determine how an object, without being a prism, can show a certain color or colors. When an object that is not a prism is struck by white light and does not radiate color on its own, why do we nevertheless see it in color? Why does something appear to be red or green or blue? This can be best understood by the process of absorption and reflection.

In this dual process, we obtain all the elements of coloration. Take, for instance, the absolutes of color, white and black. White and black are in actuality the polarities of light and darkness. As Newton stated, white light contains all the colors, and black may be defined as the absence of light. In a broader sense, however, when light includes *all* vibrations (that is, also darkness), there might be a reverse universe of "light" vibrations yet dark as black holes (collapsing stars). However, to better understand the concept of reflection and absorption in regard to color, we should first look at these functions in terms of black and white and their heat distribution.

We commonly apply the process of absorption and reflection by utilizing dark- and light-colored materials: Black is the total absorption of all colors, and white the total reflection. We experience these as coolness and heat, and we choose our clothing accordingly. If we wear dark attire during the summer months, our bodies will absorb substantial amounts of heat from the sun. This is why we commonly switch to lighter colors that reflect the heat in summer. In winter we do the opposite, wearing darker colors that absorb and hold body heat. We instinctively regulate body heat using the natural process of the absorption (black) and reflection (white) of light at the ends of the visible spectrum.

Similarly, the color of an object is also a result of its absorption and reflection of light. When light reaches the surface of an object, some but not necessarily all of the color rays are absorbed into the object. The colors visible to our eyes are those that are reflected *away* from the object. For instance, a red apple absorbs almost all colors *except* red. The fact that it reflects red means that the apple appears red to us.

How Wavelengths Determine Vibrations

Due to the absorptive and reflective process, we feel that some colors are "warmer" than others. This can best be made clear by the wavelengths of the two color rays at each end of the visible spectrum (Diagram 1-5). The violet end has shorter wavelengths, which vibrate more rapidly and have greater energy than the color rays on the red end of the spectrum. As a result, violet is tuned more to the energy of white light (acceleration, reflection) and red more to the black or "dark light" energies (absorption). Therefore, we feel that reds are warmer (which are more absorptive) than blues (more reflective).

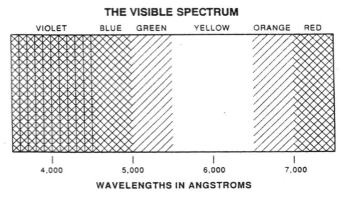

THE VISIBLE SPECTRUM

VIOLET   BLUE   GREEN   YELLOW   ORANGE   RED

4,000   5,000   6,000   7,000

WAVELENGTHS IN ANGSTROMS

Diagram 1-5. The 49th octave and its rainbow colors.

In a sunset we may also see the process of reflection and absorption at work, at least as current theory understands it. Here, dispersion or scattering of certain color rays are more of a factor than absorption. Therefore, the violet end of the spectrum (shorter wavelengths) are more dispersed by the atmosphere of the earth than the red end (longer wavelengths) at sunset.

At high noon, when the sun is above us, the pure white light comes through and causes the crisp shadows that we see then. As the sun moves farther and farther from a 90° penetration of the atmosphere (the shortest distance), it reaches the horizon at day's end, where its rays must penetrate a maximum distance through the earth's atmosphere. The shorter wavelengths of the violet spectrum are dispersed more rapidly, leaving the longer red waves for us to see and admire. This, so the theory goes, creates the reddish hues of sunset.

How Colors and Body-Energy Vibrations Interact

A color vibration is sensed not only through vision, but in many other ways. Every color vibration has an impact on all physical systems and organs of the body, which respond to these frequencies. All organisms, cells and atoms exist as energy, and each form has its frequency, or vibration — *is* energy. All energy is also either positive, negative or neutral. Color medicine and The 49th Vibrational Technique utilize these different characteristics of the colors: red (electric positive) for its stimulating effects; blue (electric negative) for its sedating effects; and green (neutral) for its ability to balance. Similarly, the various organs of the body possess functions of sedation, stimulation or neutralization through their characteristic frequencies. When the various parts of the body deviate from these expected normal vibrations, one can assume that the body is either diseased or is at least not functioning properly.

Health or lack thereof can be determined by detecting these normal or subnormal vibrations — for example, in life-energy photographs. Through vibratory corrections, the energy system can be fine-tuned and returned to a healthy state by an appropriate use of color medicine. How is this accomplished? Colors or energy vibrations, when applied to the human body — or more specifically to the human aura (the subtle energy that surrounds the physical body) — can return the entire body (or specific organs) to normal health in a very short time. It is understood, of course, that the applied vibrations will match the energy-frequency needs of an organ in terms of sedation, activation or neutralization.

To restore the proper levels of energy to the physical and etheric bodies, The 49th Vibrational Technique uses the seven rainbow colors of the spectrum: red, orange, yellow, green, blue, indigo and violet, as well as five additional colors derived from these seven, for a repertory of twelve. These twelve colors have been tested by Dinshah P. Ghadiali, and others for more than 80 years with great success. Part of that success is because the seven colors of the rainbow greatly stimulate the seven major chakras of the body (see "Recognizing the Aura and What It Can Reveal," Chapter 2). The chakras are areas of highly concentrated energy that are connected to various locations, mainly along the spinal cord. The other five colors obviously relate to important minor chakras (according to B.E.E.M. research). Understanding this relationship of the chakras to their accurately matched color frequencies makes this system more successful than other color-healing systems. Later chapters will show the relation between the unique major chakra qualities and the seven major colors of the chromatherapy healing process. They will also give a more in-depth description of how these subtle-energy fields work and how they affect the body.

Modern Interest in Frequency Therapy, or Color Medicine

The primal concepts of light therapy that are incorporated into The 49th Vibrational Technique originated in ancient cultures in India, China and Egypt. These teachings are now gaining worldwide attention from practitioners interested in drugless (metaphysical, that is) energy practices. Much of the ancient chromatherapy knowledge was advanced to its present state by Dr. Dinshah P. Ghadiali, a physician from India who spent most of his professional life researching and applying what he called Spectro-Chrome-Metry. He came to the United States in 1911, healing countless so-called hopeless cases. Many of the ideas presented in this book are a direct result of his dedicated efforts — as well as those of his son, Darius Dinshah, President of the Dinshah Health Society — to help humankind.

Dinshah had a special understanding of color medicine. Not only did he recognize the necessity of attunement of the healing colors with the chakras, but he also realized that by using the visible spectrum only, there could be no harmful effects. Colors and other vibrations continually surround us, penetrating our bodies even though in many instances we cannot see or relate to them with our physical eyes or other senses. Since some of these vibrations are beneficial and some are not, The 49th Vibrational Technique works exclusively with vibrations in the beneficial range — the 49th octave — thus healing the body, the emotions and the mind.

This therapy isolates and accentuates various colors of the spectrum and their corresponding vibrations, applying them to ailing parts of the aura and the body to restore emotions as well as damaged cells, tissues or restricted energy flows through the systematic methods provided in this book. As Dinshah discovered, color also basically represents chemical potencies at higher octaves of vibrations that affect the functioning of each system or organ in the body. There is a unique color or energy vibration that either sedates or stimulates the stream of energy through a specific organ, causing a natural biochemical reaction. Thus The 49th Vibrational Technique can heal not only the energy body (aura/emotions) by the *energy properties* of colors, but also the physical body by the colors' *chemical properties* (see Color Chemistry, Chapter 3).

When the color/element balance (energies) within the body is distorted, diseases such as cancer, diabetes, tumors, arthritis or problems related to the skin, heart and the circulatory system (to name a few) can occur. All of these common dis-eases (or disorders, as the medical profession calls them) are given treatments that often cause side effects, which may be reversed through the use of colored-light therapy if they have not reached extreme degeneration. This inexpensive yet highly effective color process — with no apparent risk — is of increasing interest to modern society.

Color Medicine for Addictions, Obesity, Allergies and Detoxification

Color therapy simply offers specific colors or levels of vibrations to specific parts of the body to regenerate and rejuvenate areas that are diseased or obesed — that is, having blocked or restricted energy. The 49th Vibrational Technique matches the specific vibrations of the colors with the needs of the specific organs or emotions in the body, enabling them to vibrate properly again. Oftentimes the body needs only a slight additional input of one or more of these color vibrations that are out of sync due to poor diet, excessive tension, toxins, anxiety or improper care of the body.

Thus color medicine can also help to eliminate dependency on addictive substances such as drugs and alcohol. It is effective in raising the metabolism of the body in order to control weight. Proper application can eliminate lung congestion, correct high levels of cholesterol and balance thyroid over- or underactivity. It can reverse much of the damage done by cigarettes or even asbestos if it has not gone beyond a certain level.

Additionally, The 49th Vibrational Technique can ease or eliminate the suffering from allergies, hayfever, colds, cataracts, diseases of the skin or gums and insomnia. The process can help to replace and strengthen thinning hair, improve the sexual organs, regulate the menstrual cycle, eliminate constipation, diarrhea and headaches, control leukemia and bleeding injuries, and repair damaged skin due to burns or cuts, leaving only a few scars in the process.

The system is effective in removing most toxins from the body, even such highly poisonous chemicals as arsenic, lead, DDT or Agent Orange. In general, the process can stimulate the immune system in the body, which in turn can control and reverse hundreds of diseases in the process. What is the underlying mechanism of this process?

Anabolism — Catabolism — Metabolism

The human body functions in two basic ways, technically referred to as anabolism and catabolism. **Anabolism** is the function of restoring, strengthening or building up the human body. **Catabolism** deals with eliminating waste products and toxic materials from the body. The healthy body can function properly only when there is a balance between these two processes (**metabolism**).

Chromatherapy is premised on the theory that the red/yellow rays, when applied to the appropriate part(s) of the body, generally stimulate the anabolic functions by which, for example, red maintains or builds the number of red blood cells and activates the liver. On the other hand, the blue/violet rays activate the catabolic aspect — for instance, in the spleen — where the older red blood cells are eliminated and white blood cells are produced. This has the effect of reinforcing the immune system, counterbalancing bacteria, etc. Thus, in color medicine red stimulates the liver (anabolic aspect) and violet stimulates the spleen (catabolic aspect). Anabolism (red) and catabolism (violet) together define metabolism (green).

One aspect of metabolic function is digestion, which is activated by yellow and sedated by blue, leaving green as their combination in the middle. Green — found in the center of the color spectrum between red/violet or yellow/blue — stimulates the pituitary gland, the master gland that controls the other glands. Green also balances the opposing forces of anabolism and catabolism (or liver and spleen) to harmonize metabolism.

The Three Basic Colors: Red, Green and Violet

Three distinct color shades or vibrations used in The 49th Vibrational Technique are Red, Green and Violet, which Dinshah called the primary colors because they create white when placed together and rotated on a disc. The other nine healing colors were all derived mathematically on the basis of their relation to, and accord with, these three primary healing colors.

Even more importantly, these basic colors are also in perfect harmony with energy centers in the body (chakras; see Chapter 2): The lowest (first) chakra corresponds with Red, the middle chakra with Green, and the highest (seventh) chakra with Violet. When these (or all) chakras are balanced, they should create a white energy field surrounding the body (aura), the same way the basic colors together create white.

This shows that the 49th vibrational system of color medicine, when used properly, harmonizes perfectly with the subtle body of man. Chromatherapy systems based on other color shades or vibrations are simply not as well researched nor as effective.

When working with pigments (paints), however, red, yellow and blue are known as the primary colors because they cannot be achieved by mixing the other colors. They cannot be used as basic vibrations (or primary colors) for color healing because they are not precisely tuned to the balance of man's energy centers and aura.

We see that Dinshah's three primary healing colors are the key to harmonizing the life energy within the human body precisely and rapidly. If properly used in conjunction with the other nine color derivatives, as described herein, they can eliminate the need for most chemical ingestions and injections (with the possible exception of emergencies), creating no harm in the process.

2

Color Energetics

How Color Medicine Interacts with the Subtle-Energy Fields of the Body

Subtle-Energy Fields and Their Movement in the Body

Humans are capable of perceiving movement of energy around or through the body, which can also be observed and even measured at both atomic and subatomic levels — for example, body temperature and brain waves. People have been trained to sense and control these energies by the use of biofeedback instruments; however, few humans are as sensitive as animals. Many birds have a so-called sixth sense, especially migratory birds, and can perceive magnetic fields in the earth (ley lines). They sense frequencies of either ultrasound or electromagnetism, permitting them to navigate great distances.

Not many humans realize that we are in fact made up of two "bodies": the gross physical body, which is perceivable by the five normal senses, and the etheric body (aura), which is often described as the ghost or higher-energy template of our physical body. This higher-energy blueprint surrounds all physical matter, or denser forms of energy. The body's bioelectrical auric response can now be scientifically documented with Tesla-Kirlian photographs.

Those who are either unaware of Tesla-Kirlian life-energy photographs or are skeptical of the existence and power of the etheric body need only look at a husband and wife who have lived together many years. They often take on some of the same physical traits and mannerisms, as well as similar emotional and thought patterns. By living in close proximity, their auras (energy fields) interact, becoming attuned and interwoven with one another.

Fields of energy react with each other in a stimulating, equalizing or sedating way. We can often experience this upon entering a room filled. with people, quickly sensing whether that room is permeated with vibrations that are harmonious or discordant. These vibrations emanate mainly from the mind and the etheric body (emotions). With our finer forces (auras) we can also sense if the vibrations in our environment feel good, bad or indifferent to us. The aura, integral to human beings, also surrounds animals, plants and all material objects, causing all things to affect one another. The energies in undisturbed nature (contrary to many cultural settings) are generally in harmony. When we travel to the country on weekends, for example, we can immediately feel the soothing and healing effects of the balanced rural energy radiating from the plant life and bodies of water. In such a setting our energy field becomes harmonized first, and then harmonizes our bodies.

The Health Aura, Sustainer of the Body

The wider aura, usually extending about one yard (one meter) from the body, functions as a shield that protects the physical, vulnerable structure. It is able to sense its surroundings in space and time and can become imbalanced by unbeneficial influences in the environment, in food or from emotions or thoughts. The aura has the ability to rebalance itself naturally. However, under unnatural conditions the imbalances may become longstanding, finally diseasing the body.

A special layer of the aura, the etheric sheath, extending only about half an inch or more (2 or more centimeters) beyond the body, can be seen as the energy mold that develops and sustains the physical body (Diagram 2-1).

The state of this etheric body ultimately determines the health of the physical body. This is demonstrated when certain energies (for example, high-frequency toxic radiation) bombard the aura. They first damage the health aura (as seen on Tesla-Kirlian photographs) and may eventually produce cancer or some other material change in the physical body. Exposure to such detrimental energies from nuclear radiation or from pesticides, herbicides and other toxic sources often does not produce immediate symptoms, as it takes time for these negative energies to penetrate the health aura and then the physical body — except when extremely high amounts are involved. This means that toxins in general weaken the etheric body first, before the physical body is affected.

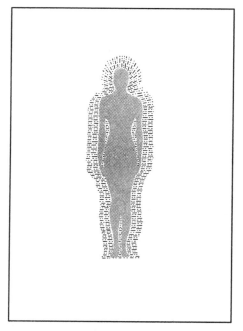

Diagram 2-1. The etheric sheath, or health aura. This sheath is a layer of the wider aura, which becomes finer and less dense the farther away it is from the body surface.

The health aura may change decades before signs of disease in the physical body become evident, because it is in the aura that disease starts and must be initially healed. Both healing and disease processes can be scientifically observed and monitored through Tesla-Kirlian photographs.

To summarize: All dis-ease begins basically in the denser part of the etheric body, in the health aura. We gain control of the ultimate health of our bodies by taking care of that sphere of energy. It is for this reason that the colored rays of The 49th Vibrational Technique are applied to the bare skin, that is, the area of the health aura (see Chapter 4 for applications).

The Four Stages of Distorted Health Auras

In order to maintain good health, the body's organs must resonate with the entire human organism as well as with the wave patterns of the universe. When an alien or destabilizing energy touches our energy field, four things can potentially happen (B.E.E.M. research):

1. Healthy Response: If the disturbing influence comes from outside and the body or specific organs are strong enough, they will either reflect away the alien vibration or entrain it to its own energy, eventually neutralizing it.

2. Cleansing: When the destabilizing vibration, of either emotional or physical origin, distorts the energy flow of the body even temporarily (at least in a specific part of the body), an illness results. This illness is a cleansing activity of the automatic balancing processes. These are often discharging or feverish illnesses.

3. Chronic Disorder: The alien or inappropriate vibration disrupts or blocks the energy flow over longer periods of time, indicating that there are internal resonating frequencies that do not allow automatic balancing. This leads to chronic disease, often lacking clear symptoms.

4. Degeneration: When the above process continues and there is no avenue of outward discharge, and emotions and beliefs increasingly support those frequencies, other parts of the body may become involved. Degenerative disease results, disharmonizing more and more areas, sometimes moving as rapidly as cancer or A.I.D.S.

These four stages of distorted, or dis-eased, auric energy have been documented on Tesla-Kirlian life-energy photographs (B.E.E.M. research and evaluation, a precise system). In all cases studied, color medicine of the 49th vibration had beneficial results when toxins were first removed from the environment and when the disease had not progressed beyond repair.

The Bonding Force of Creation: Polarity

What holds together two such different bodies as the etheric energy body and the dense physical body? This of course is also a crucial question for all matter existing in the universe. The bonding, balancing force between and within all forms of energy and matter is clearly the polarity of positive and negative. This is true for the atom, the earth, the stars and all of creation. The energies of even magnetism and gravity, which move through and around our bodies (as well as the atomic energy of matter within our bodies), follow, from a certain perspective, the same law of polarity. The cells (and all matter) are simply energy scaled down in density or lowered in vibration, in perfect balance with the whole.

From this point of view there can be no positive without a negative. There can be no cosmic activity going upward that does not cause a downward movement. Therefore our two bodies (physical and etheric) also represent the two poles – those of atomic and subatomic matter – and are bonded by polarity, as polarity is expressed everywhere in creation. Polarity, however, is not an absolute but a relative state. That is, one state can be positive to another state, yet negative to another. In other words, polarity is simply a relationship. Examples of polarities are given in the table on the next page:

Polarity is inherent in all existence and makes existence possible – at least when viewed from a three-dimensional reality. Thus existence in all its variety is merely based on different interacting densities of polarity, as our physical body (slower energy) is a manifestation of its etheric counterpart (faster energy), both directed by still higher sources. The polarities that interact between these two bodies must create a balance at all times for health. An imbalance in one must result in an imbalance in the other, since energy flows from a bioelectric positive (electric negative, etheric body) to bioelectric negative (electric positive, physical body). That is, it flows from higher to lower energy levels – with movements also the other direction – in an attempt to create

POLARITIES		
Expression	**Corresponding Opposites (poles)**	
	Physically Receptive (sedative, minus pole)	**Physically Reactive** (stimulative, plus pole)
Color	Blue (fast waves)	Red (slow waves)
Magnetism	North-seeking pole	South-seeking pole
Electricity	Electric negative	Electric positive
Bioelectricity	Bioelectric positive	Bioelectric negative
Gender	Female	Male
pH Value	Sedation by alkalinity (pH above 7)	Stimulation by acidity (pH under 7)
Chinese symbolism	Yin	Yang
Element	Oxygen	Hydrogen
Music	Slow rhythm	Fast rhythm

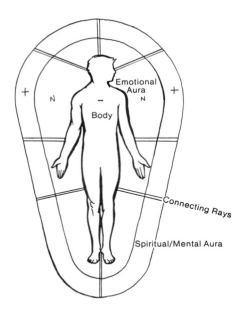

Diagram 2-2. Ideal aura/body polarity. Plus (+) denotes the spiritual/mental aura: bioelectric plus (electric minus). Neutral (N) signifies the emotional aura: bioelectric neutral (electric neutral). Minus (-) indicates the physical body: bioelectric minus (electric plus). Note that the emotional aura is ideally neutral (that is, at peace).

perfect balance (see Diagram 2-2). Within each person the energy transmitted from the etheric body finds its way into the denser subatomic matter (physical body), moved by the forces of attraction or repulsion (polarity). Likes repulse and unlikes attract, as do the poles of magnets. With this mechanism we have the means to balance (that is, heal) many disorders, or imbalances.

The Unified Field Theory/Polarity of Magnetism

Although polarity appears to be the basis of all that is created, the inquisitive mind of man extends further: The search for a unified field such as Einstein was looking for is evidence of the desire to understand what ties all creation together, including its polarities. Since all creation seems to depend on polarity for its existence, the "existence" of a unified field in terms of the three-dimensional world is a contradiction in itself. For it is a field that could have no polarity and can only exist "outside" creation — that is, in noncreated or "nonexistent" realms (where there is no polarity). This is called a *monopole field* in modern science, reminding us of the ancient Hebrew belief in two aspects of God: "deus absconditus," the unknowable God before creation (monopole field); and the "other" God, the God of creation who divided himself into polarities.

Yet in all matters relating to energy and its physical expression, the idea of polarity is the key to balancing the positive and negative forces. We therefore speak of electromagnetism and can see how this effectively works by using magnets on the body for controlling energy. Parts of the human body that are exposed to the bioelectric negative end of a magnet (north-seeking pole, blue) will, for instance, after extended periods of time, have less energy and be less active but more relaxed. If it is necessary to restrict activity, the north-seeking pole is used, for example in infections and cancer. The south-seeking pole of a magnet reinforces — unlike color medicine — both healthy and unhealthy growths. However, when noncancerous humans, animals and plants have been exposed to the bioelectric negative energies of a magnet (south-seeking pole, red), in time their systems are totally recharged. We see that the application of magnetic plus or minus poles for healing depends on the specific case: Both polarities have their important place in creating balance and restoring health.

Consequently, magnetism and The 49th Vibrational Technique basically influence our coarse physical body by harmonizing its polarities through the etheric body. The energy changes will influence the unhealthy tissues of the physical body and heal them. This is similar to acupuncture treatments, where energy vibrations are activated or sedated at or near the surface of the physical body and eventually influence the deeper levels of the physical organs.

Electromagnetic Effects on the Physical and Etheric Bodies

Since electromagnetic energy (aura) and healthy cell energy are similar in certain respects to that of magnetic poles, they will either attract or repel each other, as they cannot be all neutral as a system. Since electromagnetic movement throughout our bodies is a major factor in how well our mind, our nervous system and our organs work, it is through changing or adjusting the electromagnetic charges that light therapy produces its beneficial effect. Electromagnetic energy can be moved through our auras into the physical body by light frequencies (color), using our unique, coordinated system of twelve colors.

One can better understand how this energy works when experimenting with a television set. The set consists of a receiver, transmitter, and conductor for the electromagnetic energy. When we touch the antenna of a television set, the reception generally improves the moment our hand makes contact, because it incorporates our higher energy levels into its system. Thus it can be seen that our bodies have energy capabilities similar to the television set with its ability to transmit, receive and conduct electromagnetic or polarity forces. So it seems that our bodies are like antennas, channeling energy from higher to lower levels and vice versa (see Diagram 2-2). The energy automatically moves along the pathway (antenna) when the polarity (for example, color) is provided.

How Destructive Rays Weaken the Body

Just as improper polarity can distort the functions of a television set, so can our bodies be damaged by improper vibrations (food or drugs), especially from outside the visible spectrum (x-rays and microwaves, for example). Unfortunately, more and more of the food that is being consumed today is sterilized by irradiation to give these foods a longer shelf life. Much of this radioactive treatment (rays outside the visible spectrum) is harmful because it destroys the life energy of the food. This destructive irradiation can have serious effects on our physical bodies, such as weakening the immune system.

The same applies to microwave ovens, which use dangerous vibrations beyond the infrared range. Although there is a natural radiation of cosmic energy of different frequencies toward the earth outside the visible spectrum, it is filtered through the earth's atmosphere, so that high levels of microwaves or x-rays, for example, are unnatural on the earth's surface. Consequently, earth life has had no need to develop a defense against such rays. This is why irradiated foods and other vibrations from harmful man-made frequencies can cause long-term detrimental side effects on all life forms.

In other words, when we are adjusting energy levels (polarities) within our bodies, those energy vibrations should best stay within the visible color spectrum for safety reasons or utilize the harmonizing octaves of magnetic or sound healing, unless there is a very specific need to go to either the ultraviolet or infrared end of the spectrum. Harmful vibrations should be excluded during recovery, at the very least.

Since our bodies consist of constantly shifting and changing energy patterns that occasionally cause disharmony, colored light is the simple and appropriate way to correct any energy imbalance. By using only the visible light spectrum, The 49th Vibrational Technique can have no detrimental or harmful effects when administered properly, even if applied on an excessive basis (not recommended). Certain feelings or symptoms are signals to cease the session or change the vibrational rate (color). However, symptoms occurring from excessive use of colored light tend to disappear without long-standing negative effects. There is no other medium for controlling imbalanced energies (dis-ease) — whether it be conventional medicine or otherwise — that is as effective with so little chance of harmful side effects.

The Importance of Balanced Body/Mind/Emotion Polarities

Balanced polarities are necessary for the health of the entire physi-cal/emotional/mental system, which consists of bioelectric poles. The physical form has two main layers of energy around it (not considering the health aura separate here), which are the denser emotional aura and the finer mental aura (Diagram 2-2). In this system the energy of thought patterns, mental and even higher etheric layers, represents the bioelectric positive pole (electric negative). Our emotions — our way of expressing ourselves — should generally be the balancing, neutral pole of peace, whereas the dense physical matter of our body (our organs) can be classified as the bioelectric negative pole (see Diagram 2-2). Rays of energy piercing through the neutral layer (emotional aura) seem to connect the positive (mental aura) and negative (physical body) poles. If these three are out of harmony, bioelectric imbalance occurs, resulting in disease on mental, emotional and physical levels.

The neutral middle of our energy spectrum — our emotional space — can be directly affected by physical events. For instance, extreme hunger can have an almost overwhelming effect on our emotions. Our emotional body, which should ideally be calm and neutral, may then be thrown out of balance. For instance, we see hyperactivity mainly after eating too much starchy food and white sugar, which affect our emotion-al body and the physical and mental bodies as well.

Imbalances can also easily come from the nonphysical through negative thoughts and especially negative emotions (anxiety, worry, shock, jealousy, anger etc.). It is for this reason that in India spiritual students have been taught to keep their thoughts positive and their emotions neutral, at peace.

Unfortunately, many decisions are made during an emotional reac-tion to an event. As this negative energy affects the physical/men-tal/emotional harmony, it also begins to change the normal physical processes (blood pressure, heart rate and digestive functions, for example). As the process continues, it becomes aggravated and finally depletes the system. The nervous energy and tension then tend to seek immediate balance, unfortunately believed to be attained through such stimulants as excessive drinking of coffee and alcohol, poor diet (refined sugar and flour, animal fats and animal protein) or inadequate physical conditioning. Such an effect can only be temporary and will finally deplete the bioelectric system. The way we treat our bodies by the foods we eat, the toxins we contact or inhale, the exercise or lack thereof, may each have the overall effect of disrupting the energies of our body/mind/emotion system.

By simply looking at ourselves (without judging) on mental, emotional and physical levels and recognizing our shortcomings — whether self-induced or a result of our poisoned environment — we can begin to make corrections through the use of the appropriate color vibrations that counteract the imbalances. However, even when we are not aware of what needs healing in our systems, the colors for one symptom may also heal what is unnoticed in other areas or on other levels, by their multilevel balancing effects.

The Polarity of Colors

In color therapy the ultraviolet or blue end of the spectrum resembles, in effect, the electric negative side, and the red or infrared end the electric positive side. The color green and its vibrations are neutral and harmonize electromagnetic polarity. Electromagnetic effects are also involved in the acid/alkaline balance in the body. High acid levels generally cause inflammation, swelling and fever, duplicating the effects of excessive red vibrations in the body. In this case the blue colors are given for balance. High alkaline levels — too much blue in the body — are sedating, which can result in an overrelaxed condition. Here warm colors are given for stimulation. When the two poles (red/acidic, blue/ alkaline) are in balance, we have a well-functioning polarity, such as when oxygen (O) (blue) and hydrogen (H) (red) combine to form H_2O (water), which is neutral and in its flow slightly alkaline — as the body should be.

To further understand the effects of color, one can consider the use of hot and cold compresses. Heat is stimulating, as is the red end of the color spectrum, and draws activity (blood) to an area. Heat, for instance, draws blood flow to the body surface and nutrients are thus supplied to the cells. On the other hand, cool temperatures (the blue end of the visible spectrum) have a tendency to calm and comfort an area, relieving swellings and driving the blood deeper into the tissues.

In the polarity of color we thus receive an extremely effective tool to stimulate, sedate or neutralize imbalanced energy in the body and aura layers (the three-body system).

Recognizing the Aura and What It Can Reveal

Since the body is a product of the energy mold or aura, inside which the body originally grew, the aura tells the story of each organ, cell or molecule to those who are capable of reading it. The aura unfolds our purposes and goals in life, our frustrations and, for our purposes, our state of health. As the patterns of our personalities change, we can monitor the progress or lack thereof, determine if we have missed or used opportunities. Although the long-term vibration of the personality is in the aura, our current state of being is readily visible as well. How can the aura tell us all this incredible information? It speaks to us through its many vibrations, expressed as colors. We have only to learn how to read it.

The aura, although surrounding the entire body, is most evident around the head and shoulders due to master glands and major nervous connections located there. Mind and emotions are likely to be the governing factors that determine the colors in the aura; however, the environment can also play a part. Most colors in the aura are constantly changing and are a blend representing temporary or permanent imbalance. A perfect aura would probably be pure white, resulting from the perfect balance of the seven main chakra colors (see Diagram 2-3) — since their perfectly balanced rainbow colors appear white when rotated on a disk. The chakras are the seven main energy fields related to the major organs in the body.

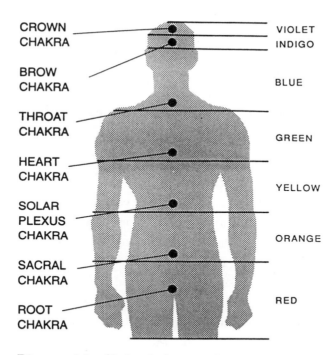

Diagram 2-3. Chakra/color coordination. How The 49th Vibrational Technique colors correspond to the chakra system and various parts of the body.

Anyone can now see the auric responses with equipment such as a Tesla-Kirlian device. It can record one's present condition by merely photographing the hands or feet. However, with proper training one can see the aura directly and read others' strengths and weaknesses, their health patterns, their talents or misfortunes and even predict approaching death. More important, we also can learn to see or sense our own aura, enabling us to heal ourselves.

We often sense the aura of others quite well when we say, "That color doesn't suit you" or "That color is just right for you." In both instances we are reading the color needs and comparing them subconsciously with the person's aura and clothing. Colors one wears often reflect unconscious choices for balancing one's energies, when feeling or intuition determines the choice. The color needs of the aura can be partly furnished by the color of one's garments. Faster and more effective, however, is the application of electromagnetic light vibrations (colored light).

Color Meanings and Tonal Equivalents

Just as the states of physical organs and systems are expressed in vibrations/color (for each color/chakra, refer to Diagram 2-3), so are emotions and thoughts. Consequently the colors of the aura tell us about the personality in its present state. Since Dinshah scientifically correlated and formulated musical notes to the colors, we provide here the meaning of colors and their musical equivalents.

RED: Correlating musical note, **G**. Red in the aura indicates a physical and more materialistic orientation, with a strong concern for physical life (predominance of the root chakra). It shows a vigorous, active, forceful person, often with a warm and affectionate nature, yet impulsive and passionate; may be domineering or angry.

There may be courage, passionate love, hatred and revenge. Red in the aura may indicate a low energy level and problems with the nervous system. The brighter, lighter and clearer the red, the warmer and more generous the person. The darker the red, the more impulsive the person; even malice may show.

1. Bright, clear red: Pride, generosity, positive ambition
2. Dark red: Anger
3. Ruddy dark red: Sensuality
4 Cloudy dark red: Cruelty
5. Pink: Often seen in children and spiritual adults, a sign of love and vitality

ORANGE: Correlating musical note, **A**. A clear orange indicates that a person is thoughtful and considerate of others, vital and healthy, with a certain dominance in the second chakra. The more reddish tones point to selfishness and pride. Certain shades of orange can also indicate kidney problems.

1. Clear orange-gold: Vitality, health, self-control, consideration, balance
2. Reddish orange: Pride, selfishness
3. Brownish orange: Low intellect, lacking ambition

YELLOW: Correlating musical note, **A#**. Golden yellow indicates a

system. Although our minds can block out certain sounds or v
our bodies at the cellular level cannot. Our physical bodie
mersed in an ocean of vibrations that include unheard sound that may
cause stress, tension and disease from an unrecognized source.

Modern society, being basically visual, places less emphasis on
sound than sight. Much evidence has accumulated, however, that sound
can not only harm but also heal. To create sounds in tune with the
healing lights and the aura, we must use a harmonious formula that
reduces color frequencies to sound levels for a more powerful, synergis-
tic effect.

Cymatics: Combining Sound and Light
to Work on Energy Blockage

A tuning fork, when placed near undamped piano strings, will cause
– or entrain – a sympathetic resonance in those strings of the same or
related frequency. When it is understood what "sound" (frequency) a
healthy organ emits, then that same sound (frequency) transmitted to the
unhealthy organ will tend to entrain it, causing it to resonate once more
at its natural frequency. However, results with sound are not a function
of volume (amplitude, or quantity) but pitch (frequency, quality), similar
to the effect of color in color medicine, where the intensity (quantity) of
the light source is not as important as is the color frequency (quality).

Therefore, The 49th Vibrational Technique suggests a formula
outlined by Dinshah that reduces mathematically the higher vibrations –
found in the twelve healing colors – to the frequencies of audible sound
(see Chapter 4).

The colors we use vibrate in the visible spectrum (the 49th octave)
between 397 trillion (red) and 665 trillion (violet) times per second.
Human hearing ranges roughly between 16 and 16,000 cycles per second
in the 4th to 15th octaves. The medium range of human hearing is the
9th octave, 40 octaves below visible light. The higher (faster) frequencies of the visible spectrum enable light to penetrate all levels of
existence more effectively than sound with its slower (grosser) frequencies. Light works primarily on the etheric level and is stronger and more

effective by itself than sound. Sound therapy works more on a physical scale, yet may still treat energy blockages through the cells and the spinal cord. However, together light and sound can synergistically reinforce each other to create improved health.

We might compare the combined healing process of attuned light and sound to the use of three tuning forks. Three matching forks (representing color, sound and body cells) are tuned to the same pitch. When one of them is struck, the others vibrate in resonance with the first. Similarly, by fine-tuning two body organs to vibrate harmoniously through sound and/or light, the tissues between them will also reflect this movement of new energy, freeing themselves from blockages or disease in the process.

Orchestra of Life: Attunement to the Green Earth Cycle

We may compare the body with a full-scale orchestra where each instrument (organ) vibrates at the frequency natural to it and in harmony with the vibrations of all other instruments. We also find such a "tuned orchestra" between man and nature: In a relaxed state (for example, in meditation), the human brain (cerebrum) vibrates at a rate of 7 to 8 cycles per second (alpha state). The entire body is then relaxed and receptive to healing when the cerebrum reaches that range. Perhaps not surprisingly, the earth also vibrates at about 8 cycles per second, which results from the speed of the electromagnetic radiance divided by the circumference of the earth.

This earth frequency corresponds to that of Dinshah's Green (B.E.E.M. research), which balances too-rapid or too-slow processes of organs. No wonder that all life forms possessing nervous systems are attuned to this relaxing green earth frequency. Our hypothetical orchestra (the body) both emits and responds to this 8-cycle frequency. Within the human system (as in the orchestra), each component, with its unique tonal quality, plays its own notes. Just as the violin has a tonal quality and thematic contribution different from that of the flute, so has the heart vibration compared to that of the spleen. Yet they all play harmoniously in concert with each other.

Prior to tuning up, the orchestral instruments may be off-key, as are the body organs from time to time. A hit-or-miss approach to fine-tuning the instruments cannot work in either the orchestra or in the human body. By introducing finely tuned vibrations of color — as harmonious as the earth cycle — The 49th Vibrational Technique can help heal the body without destructive side effects.

Tapes with harmonious sounds for each color may be made to accompany colored light therapy, wherein the exact reduction formula is obviously of overall importance (see Chapter 4).

Effects of Monochord/Color and Rhythm on the Body

Greek musicians recognized that even a single note, called a monochord, can affect man and beast. They were able to sense the tone that represented the key to a particular individual's state of perfect health, and by constantly playing this note on a flute, heal that person. Eastern religions do this through mantras with several single-tone sequences.

The monochord approach of The 49th Vibrational Technique, similar to that of the Greeks, works on the higher as well as the grosser (physical) levels of life energy to effect healing. Since we are using a direct reduction formula to translate the visible to the audible range, we correlate reds (stimulating) to lower sounds (slower frequencies) and blues (sedating) to higher ones (faster frequencies).

It is well-known that a rapid beat or quick-moving melody stimulates the nervous system and slower rhythms and melodies can induce restful sleep and a peaceful mind. It is not yet fully understood why slower *color vibrations* (red) stimulate but slower *rhythms* sedate.

When one focuses attention within one's body in quiet surroundings, one can feel rhythmic sounds moving through the body. A simple humming exercise can demonstrate how various sound waves produce different effects in the body — like the various vibrations of color therapy. Through the proper use of color/sound therapy, the nervous system and the entire three-body system can again dance to a harmonious energy tune.

The Interplay Between Music and the Chakra System

To make the monochord sound more interesting, we support additional orchestral instruments to accompany the monochord, from the gentle woodwind to the more rhythmic drums. Interestingly, in music the word for this variety is "color," denoting the vastly different feel contributed by each different instrument's tonal quality. In The 49th Vibrational Technique sound design, in which pitch is correlated to color, a special rhythm is also of significance in terms of the healing process, for it is the rhythmic patterns that assist in opening the seven chakras. A soft type of jazz is said to open the 6th and 7th chakras; soft rock and heavy metal sounds appeal to the root and sacral chakras; and reggae opens up the middle chakras (3rd, 4th, and 5th). (See Diagram 2-3.)

The 49th Vibrational Technique sound designs — using the proper monochords — are played with seven different instruments that work on the chakras. The third eye is stimulated first with buzzing sounds, then the sounds focus on each chakra from the root chakra to the crown. Each tape, with a basic monochord sound, relates to a single color. For example, a synthesizer focuses on middle C (green on the color spectrum) for one hour with seven instrumental tonal qualities for opening the seven chakras.

Colors	Chakras	Tone (Monochord)	Instrumental Sounds	Rhythms
Red	Root	G	Crickets	Soft Rock
Orange	Sacral	A	Harp	Soft Rock
Yellow	Solar Plexus	A#	Wooden flute	Reggae
Green	Heart	C	Bells/Drums	Reggae
Blue	Throat	D	Ocean waves	Reggae
Indigo	Brow	D#	Bees/Buzzing insects	Jazz
Violet	Crown	E	Om sound/	Jazz

Color/Chakra/Sound Correlations

People in many countries traditionally use music for healing. Accomplished musical groups playing classical compositions of Bach, Beethoven, Vivaldi, Mozart and Handel may vibratorily lead through all chakras, clearing each in the process. That is why this music has survived the test of time. The seven chakras and their corresponding sounds, instruments or rhythms are as follows.

Harmonious music therapy, when supplementing chromatherapy, is like an intravenous feeding — noninvasive, however — energizing without one's conscious attention. Sound is a carrier wave to the subconscious, a vital link to a holistic healing program. It is interesting to see that acute disorders (with sharp pain or fever) seem to call for cool colors (faster frequencies) but slower rhythms; and chronic diseases (without fever but with rigidity) for warmer colors (slower frequencies) but faster rhythms.

The 49th Vibrational Technique — *Auric-Frequency Precision Is Its Secret*

As man is a complex being, healing often appears complicated. Man's nervous system, having developed over millions of years, is far more detailed than any electric wiring system that humans could ever devise. This nervous system, more sophisticated than the most advanced computer system in the world, consists of branches and synapses of bioelectric and electromagnetic fields. It carries varying currents and charges and is capable of retrieving, storing and transmitting incredible amounts of information.

When even those trained in modern medicine cannot fully comprehend how a human being bends his fingers, how can they understand how the body actually heals itself? The simple movement of a finger, which we do quite subconsciously through a series of electromagnetic impulses, remains unexplained. These generating impulses are a product of our higher selves, related to our subtle-energy fields. Subtle energy is heightened consciousness with an inherent wisdom that works toward the best for the whole. When provided with precisely the right vibration, it can heal itself and the physical body. Thus when illness occurs, the insertion of a frequency (color), reinforced by correlating sound frequencies, can bring balance back into the life-energy field and the body.

Color medicine is simple, but it is highly effective *because* it uses the body's own wisdom; its simplicity is, in fact, the key to its effectiveness, networking beyond the conscious mind, within the subconscious.

Many know that the secret to success in life is not, contrary to what has long been taught, necessarily a result of long hours and hard work. What works in life also works in color therapy: Precision is the secret. It is the exact amount of energy that is needed, no more nor less, in the right place, at the appointed time, and in the appropriate manner that gets results. In The 49th Vibrational Technique we do not deal with the physical body per se (comparable to long hours and limited results); we address with a fine-tuned precision the etheric (spiritual energy) in our system for the maximum results.

3

Color Harmonics

The Twelve Healing Colors and Their Use

Color Psychology — The Power of the Subconscious

We all have ways of expressing discomfort, in terms of color. For instance, we might be "feeling blue" or be "green with envy." Sometimes we "see red" or are "black with anger." We also know how a sunshiny day with a clear blue sky can improve our morale, whereas a cloudy, rainy day can be depressing. This becomes even more evident in the four seasons: We tend to be more inward during the late fall and winter months, which have less color outdoors, then begin to blossom out again in spring and summer, somewhat like the plants themselves. This points out the overall effect that color or energy vibrations may have on us. Every change, whether from the seasons, the weather or any other source, affects the way we think, the way we feel and the way we act.

We have little or no control over most body functions, because they arise directly from the subconscious. Such functions as respiration, blood circulation, digestion, temperature control, disease resistance and cell regeneration are automatic. There is an intricate system at work, and even the most highly educated practitioners in medicine cannot fully explain how even the human digestive system functions.

On the other hand, the so-called conscious activity of the brain/mind directs most of our physical activities, and can choose to balance this life energy. Any imbalance in one of the three bodies — the mind, for instance — can make us sick. Our thoughts are chiefly responsible for generating the negative energy associated with hatred, anger, resentment, envy, jealousy etc., which are often related to mental disorders and other malfunctions of the body. Fatigue, stress and fear are all generated by the mind-energies that disrupt the health of the body.

Since we are an open system in terms of our physical, psychological and spiritual existence, any negative energy within the mind and emotions will circulate throughout our physical structure. The negative energy finally becomes a part of one's structure when it encapsulates itself as cramps, cysts or tumors or distorts systems by its own distorted movement.

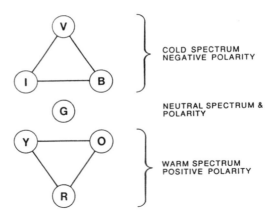

Diagram 3-1. **Rainbow colors and areas of correspondence.** This illustration indicates the main color response in the body: The reds correspond to the lower body; the green to the heart; and the blues to the upper body. (R = red; O = orange; Y = yellow; G = green; B = blue; I = indigo; V = violet.) The cold spectrum (blues) is electric negative; the warm spectrum (reds) is electric positive.

In this way the function of an organ or life-support system may deteriorate or even cease entirely. Color vibrations, when applied in an integrated system such as The 49th Vibrational Technique, can restore positive energies in both the emotions and the body systems. The energy field and the body itself absorb the needed color vibrations, and the wisdom of the subconscious mind directs them to appropriate areas for healing. Warm colors tend to activate the lower body, Green resonates mainly with the heart area, and the blue colors correspond to the upper body (Diagram 3-1), relating to the chakra colors (see Chapter 2).

Let us now look at the effects on the human system of all twelve colors utilized by The 49th Vibrational Technique.

Primary, Secondary and Tertiary Attuned Colors

The three primary colors, Red (warm), Green (neutral), and Violet (cool), create three additional or secondary colors in the color-therapy spectrum: Yellow, Blue and Magenta. These, combined with the primary colors, produce the tertiary colors: Orange, Lemon, Turquoise, Indigo, Purple and Scarlet. In our system all the secondary and tertiary colors are derived from and in tune with the vibrations of the three primary colors. Thus all twelve colors are attuned to each other and to the aura (see Diagram 3-2).

Grouping of the Healing Colors

The array of primary, secondary and tertiary colors can be divided into warm, neutral and cool colors. The warm colors are Red, Orange, Yellow and Lemon; the neutral color is Green; and the cool colors are Turquoise, Blue, Indigo and Violet. The remaining three colors — Purple, Magenta and Scarlet — are the circulatory colors drawn from vibrations of both the warm and cool spectrum.

The Healing Power of the Warm (Infra-Green) Colors

The warm colors of the spectrum (Red, Yellow, Orange and Lemon) are stimulating and detoxifying. They are, as a rule, not to be used with fevers or inflammations.

RED, a primary color, is located at one end (the infrared) of the visible spectrum. Red, which has a connotation of heat or fire, is a stimulant, and when used properly activates all five senses, the sensory nervous system, and the liver, as well as the generation of red blood platelets and hemoglobin. Red generally rejuvenates the human body by purifying the blood, but must be used with extreme caution, as it tends to purify rapidly through the skin and to activate inflammation and certain physical or emotional conditions. Red counteracts x-ray and ultraviolet burns. When a warm color (from the red end) is used on the body for a week, it needs to be balanced with one treatment from the other side of the spectrum (one of the blues). Red vibrates at 436 trillion times per second.

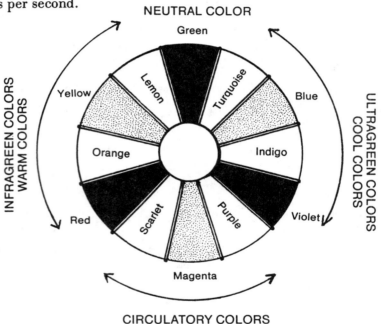

Primary Colors: Red, Green, Violet
Secondary Colors: Yellow, Blue, Magenta
Tertiary Colors: Orange, Lemon, Turquoise, Indigo, Purple, Scarlet

Diagram 3-2. Color grouping of the 12 aura-attuned colors. All twelve are used in The 49th Vibrational Technique.

ORANGE is next to Red, moving toward the center of the visible spectrum. It is produced by combining Yellow and Red glass filters. Orange boosts the energy in the lungs and stomach, even assisting vomiting, if necessary. It raises the pulse rate but not the blood pressure. This color also stimulates the thyroid and the growth of bone, producing life energy that then radiates throughout the entire body. Orange releases the energy trapped or blocked within organs (such as in cramps, congestion, flatulence), enabling it to move to other body areas. It helps heal bruises after Indigo has been used for the swelling. Orange and its vibrations have a major effect on the etheric body, and is considered an emotional uplifter. Orange vibrates at 473 trillion times per second.

YELLOW, the third color from the infrared end, is a vibrational combination of Red and Green. This secondary color is a stimulant for the sensory and motor nervous systems. Yellow tones the muscles, activates the lymph glands (which in turn cleanse the blood) and improves the digestive system, stimulating the intestines, pancreas and digestive fluids. It is considered a cleanser, and when properly applied can remove many of the toxins or parasites from the digestive tract. It clears up imperfections in the skin by stimulating the lymphatic system and acts as a purifier in the bloodstream.

Yellow, the color of the mind or intellect, can raise low-energy emotional states (depression, apathy, discouragement). Like other warm colors, it needs to be balanced by a color from the blue side once a week, as the cleansing process can sometimes cause excessive cleansing activities in the eliminative systems (diarrhea or fever). Yellow vibrates at 510 trillion times per second.

LEMON is a combination of Yellow and Green. It stimulates the colon like a mild laxative and activates the thymus gland, an important organ in the immune system. It is a bone builder and an excellent detoxifier of harsh chemicals. Therefore, Lemon is generally considered the master cleanser, as it expels toxins such as lead, DDT or arsenic rapidly through the skin and the aura. It dissolves blood clots often within hours, rejuvenates the body and in time eliminates even long-standing toxins. It nourishes and repairs cells in chronic disorders by adding mineral vibrations to the body, and it stimulates the brain. It is balanced by one of the blue colors (especially Turquoise) once a week. Lemon vibrates at 547 trillion times per second.

The Healing Power of the Neutral Color Green

When in doubt as to what color to choose because of a lack of indications, use the neutral Green. It can balance both over- or underactive conditions. Green is the master color, the middle of the spectrum. It is a tension reliever that balances the cerebrum and stimulates the pituitary gland, which controls all other glands in the body. Green is also the most predominant color of the vegetation on this planet. This balancing color builds cells and tissues, and is the stabilizing color for all dysfunctions, whether chronic or acute. Many disorders can be cleared up just by using Green alone, as an antiseptic, germicide and disinfectant, as it eliminates microorganisms and prevents decay. It is the main color used for the common cold and for relieving food poisoning and bacterial infections. When body wastes are eliminated properly, bacteria cannot live off healthy tissue. Green also builds muscle and tissue, especially when combined with Turquoise. It relieves tension and regulates the etheric body. Since Green is a neutral color, there is no need to balance it once a week. Green vibrates at 584 trillion times per second.

The Healing Power of the Cool (Ultra-Green) Colors

On the other side of the spectrum toward the ultraviolet end are the colors Turquoise, Blue, Indigo and Violet. They relieve fevers and soothe many types of pains. They are not — as a rule — to be used in cases of hypothermia (subnormal temperature) or for burns from x-rays or ultraviolet rays.

TURQUOISE (a combination of Blue and Green), is the opposite of the color Lemon. It builds the skin and is especially useful for the repair and nourishment of cells in acute disorders. When used with Green or Blue it is extremely effective for healing infections, burns and wounds. It is especially recommended for third-degree burns, used in conjunction with coconut oil after the use of Blue, to heal the skin with little or no scarring. Turquoise is cerebrally calming. It acts as a coolant upon all types of low fevers, especially for headaches and other cranial pressures. Turquoise is also an effective vibration for sound sleep (besides Blue,

Indigo, Violet and Purple) and may be used instead of sleeping pills because of its calming effect on the mind. Turquoise is balanced once a week by Lemon. It vibrates at 621 trillion times per second.

BLUE increases the elimination of toxins through perspiration, stimulates intuitive powers and is a vitality builder. It relieves the irritation and pain from burns and itching, providing more restful sleep. The oxygen ray found in Blue fills the lungs and interacts with the hydrogen ray in Red to relieve fever and inflammation. Blue activates the pineal gland; it is the color of the spirit. It is balanced once a week by one of the warm colors. Blue vibrates at 658 trillion times per second.

INDIGO is the next color of the spectrum. It is a cooling color that activates the parathyroid and calms the thyroid. It controls abscesses and relieves or eliminates discharges and bleeding, even in the brain. It also calms the respiratory system, reduces swelling and has an anesthetic effect on the body (thus is used for the relief of most pain). Indigo can improve one's emotional state by its sedative effect, and it has a generally calming, inward-turning energy vibration. It also has contractive characteristics whereby it can firm, tone and tighten up the flesh and arrest or shrink tumors, swellings and unhealthy growths. It is balanced with one of the warm colors once a week. Indigo vibrates at 695 trillion times per second.

VIOLET is the last color on the blue end and thus has the shortest wavelength of the visible colors. It has the capability to control hunger (and thus weight) through calming the metabolic process. It soothes all overactive organs of the body except the spleen. It relaxes the muscles, including the heart, and has antibiotic characteristics through stimulating the production of leukocytes, which destroy harmful bacteria. Violet builds the spleen and calms the lymphatic glands. It is also a blood purifier and helps maintain the necessary mineral balance in our bodies, as all other colors do. Calming the nerves, it is an aid to meditation and sleep. Violet may act as a pain reliever after first trying Indigo. It is balanced by one of the warm colors once a week. Violet vibrates at 731 trillion times per second.

The Healing Power of the Circulatory Colors

In addition to these nine warm, neutral and cool colors, there are three more colors in the visible spectrum that further fine-tune the energy for specific healing purposes, especially heart, kidney and circulatory functions. These three additional colors utilized in The 49th Vibrational Technique are Magenta, Purple and Scarlet (Diagram 3-2).

PURPLE (a combination of Violet and Yellow) calms the emotions as well as the activity in the arteries. It stimulates activity in the veins and relieves headaches and excessive pain from pressure by decreasing sensitivity. It lowers blood pressure and induces sleep. Purple slows down overactive kidneys and adrenalin glands and reduces sexual activity and heart rate, thus strengthening the organs when overactive and exhausted. It decreases menstrual pain and bleeding in the lungs. Purple may also be used when the heart/lung ratio calls for it (see Chapter 4). Purple can eliminate recurrent high fevers associated with such diseases as malaria and rheumatic fever. It is balanced by Scarlet once a week. Purple vibrates at 621 trillion times per second.

MAGENTA (a combination of Red and Violet) balances the emotions. It levels blood pressure, automatically raising or lowering it to normal. It balances such conditions as abnormal sex desires by combining it with Turquoise and Purple. Magenta stimulates and nourishes the kidneys, the adrenals, the heart and the circulatory system. It is also an aura builder and is similar to Green in that it can be used for most energy disorders. Magenta is a neutral color with no need to balance it once a week with another color. It vibrates at 584 trillion times per second.

SCARLET (a combination of Red and Blue) speeds up the heartbeat, stimulates the arteries and sedates the activity of the veins (the reverse of Purple). It raises the blood pressure, stimulates the kidneys and adrenals and activates the emotions by increasing sensitivity. Scarlet is a general stimulant, and also increases sluggish menstrual discharges. It can accelerate the birth process at the time of birth and is balanced by Purple once a week. Scarlet is the strongest of the twelve healing colors and needs to be used with utmost care. Scarlet vibrates at 547 trillion times per second.

The Complementary, Precisely Aura-Attuned Color Scheme

Ten of the twelve healing colors have a complementary color (see Diagram 3-3) or vibration used to balance or counterbalance their vibratory effects. It is important, in some cases, to use the exact complementary color for this purpose. If an exact counterbalance is not necessary, it is sufficient to balance warm colors with any of the cool colors — and vice versa — once in awhile. Purple is still balanced by Scarlet, and vice versa.

The 49th Vibrational Technique generally establishes a rule of seven: For every six uses of predominantly one color, a color of the opposite side of the spectrum should be used once for balance. That is, after the use of any warm color for a week, use any cool color once. The main color for counterbalancing the warm colors is Turquoise; Lemon counterbalances the cool colors. However, in extreme cleansing situations (fevers, diarrhea, rashes etc.) the exact complementary color, as given below, may be necessary. A complementary color may also be required once (or several times in some cases) that does not correspond with the color given in the schedules in the Appendix.

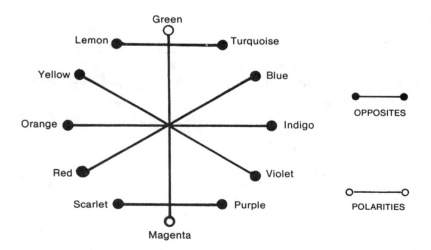

Diagram 3-3. The complementary colors. These color frequencies counterbalance each other's effects when necessary.

The complementary (opposite) colors for chromatherapy are stated as follows:

Complementary Colors		
Red	↔	Blue
Orange	↔	Indigo
Yellow	↔	Violet
Lemon	↔	Turquoise
Green	↔	no complementary color (polarity with Magenta)
Scarlet	↔	Purple

Each of the ten complementary color pairs work in opposition to each other to rebalance the energy system. Magenta and Green have no opposite because they are the fulcrum, affecting vibrations of both sides of the spectrum and equilibrating body and emotions.

Because the twelve Dinshah colors are based on three primary colors (Red, Green and Violet), Dinshah needed only five glass slides of the primary and secondary colors to create all twelve healing vibrations (see table below and Diagram 3-4). This simplicity reveals the attunement and precision of his color system. The colors are blended as follows from Red, Yellow, Green, Blue and Violet glass slides not possible with present plastic filters:

Dinshah Glass-Slide Composition			
Color	Combination	Frequency	Freq. Combination
Red	primary color (slide 1)	436	436
Orange	combine Red & Yellow	473	(436 + 510)/2 = 473
Yellow	secondary color (slide 2)	510	510
Lemon	combine Yellow & Green	547	(510 + 584)/2 = 547
Green	primary color (slide 3)	584	584
Turquoise	combine Blue & Green	621	(658 + 584)/2 = 621
Blue	secondary color (slide 4)	658	658
Indigo	combine Blue & Violet	695	(658 + 731)/2 = 695
Violet	primary color (slide 5)	731	731
Purple	combine Violet & Yellow	621 reverse	(731 + 510)/2 = 621
Magenta	combine Red & Violet	584 reverse	(436 + 731)/2 = 584
Scarlet	combine Red & Blue	547 reverse	(436 + 658)/2 = 547

Since, however, the glass slides break easily and it is difficult to reattune the replacements, durable plastic gels (filters) are recommended for tonation of the body (see Chapter 4). Thus aura attunement by colored light is always at hand.

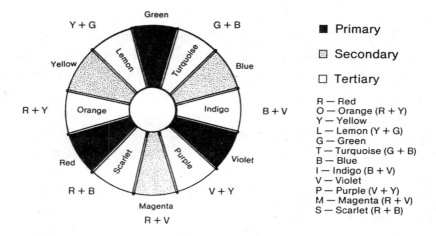

Diagram 3-4. **Dinshah color combinations.** These are the color combinations of his glass slides.

How Man's Physical and Biochemical Systems Depend on Light

Life on earth as well as throughout our solar system depends on the ultimate source of energy (light), which is the sun. Plant growth, animal development and behavior, and man's physical and biochemical systems all depend directly on light and the energy generated therefrom. We see the effects of shifting light patterns in the cycles of day and night as well as the seasons, all of which have a tremendous effect on human life. The link between the sun and life on the planet makes all living organisms (plant, animal or human) subject to the same laws of nature. The smallest cell on our planet and the largest star in the universe are governed by the same principles of energy and light.

We can see strong effects of light upon plants when they are grown in a controlled environment where, for instance, a glass cover is used for temperature control. Because glass has a tendency to screen out the ultraviolet wavelengths of light, over a relatively short time plants or vegetables that need ultraviolet rays will not grow as well as when they are covered by certain plastic substitutes. By simply moving the plants into a plastic-covered environment, they will quickly recuperate, since most plastics do not screen out ultraviolet wavelengths.

The color vibrations of the visible spectrum also have a major effect on the functions, growth and development of animals and humans. One can see this in the way animals react to light. When they are bred under conditions of natural sunlight, animals produce approximately equal numbers of female and male offspring. Under pinkish fluorescent lighting they tend to produce almost exclusively male litters (red is termed *yang*, or male, in Chinese philosophy). Those that are raised under bluish lights tend to produce almost exclusively female litters (blue is considered *yin*, or female, in the Chinese system). Whatever else these facts tell us, we can see that if a specific light vibration can influence the gender of certain animals, it is likely to have other influences on the physical organism and on emotional levels as well.

In the human being we know about the biochemical effects of light on moods, tissues and glands. Without sufficient sunlight people become moody, pale and weak. Children may not grow properly with insufficient sunlight, because the skin's secretion of vitamin D (necessary for healthy skin and bone growth) is dependent on light. Light is absorbed by the tissues (especially of the eyes) and can be transformed into body warmth or broken into light of different wavelengths, resulting in proper body chemistry.

Side Effects of Drugs versus the Safety of Color Medicine

The concept of beneficially influencing living beings through the use of appropriate light frequencies (color biochemistry) underlies the healing process in The 49th Vibrational Technique.

Many unexplained illnesses today can be directly related to the ingestion of drugs. These may relieve certain symptoms, but have mysterious and often detrimental side effects. Color medicine, when used properly, has no detrimental effects, as it does not suppress symptoms but goes directly to their cause, where energy has been either interrupted or unbalanced.

By offering the element to the body through colored light, the body can choose what and how much it needs. Color medicine, therefore, restores the energy balance without the potentially harmful effects of chemicals or drugs — which are not gently offered but forced into the digestive tract, bloodstream or tissues. As in homeopathy or acupuncture, color therapy works according to the principles of energy, not by directly affecting the organs themselves but by restoring balance to the body's etheric energy levels. The healing of the physical or denser organs soon follows. Color medicine is based on the concept that a chemical imbalance, a state of disease, and an inappropriate energy vibration in the body are all synonymous. Dis-ease basically begins when one's overall auric energy patterns deviate from white, the composite aura color. One might assume, then, that white rays would be the most effective cure, but this is not the case in a weak system. White rays can be too powerful for damaged bodies, which cannot properly sort out or select the required frequencies from the white ray and therefore need a specific, attuned healing color.

Color Medicine Contrasted with Orthodox Medicine

Since light influences the tissues in living beings by penetrating the health aura, its effects on the human body are generally classified as either direct or indirect. Orthodox medicine and science provide their own explanations of how light works. These explanations are based on strictly physical functions and ignore the bioelectric energy field, which has been demonstrated or photographed with Tesla-Kirlian devices for over 100 years.

Current scientific/medical understanding of light's effect on physical tissue is as follows:

(1) Direct: The body tissues actually absorb the charge of light, reacting in a photosynthetic process. When radiant energy is absorbed,

the energy levels are raised to a higher energy status (at least temporarily) and are able to act as catalysts for oxidation and for combining numerous compounds before returning to the normal energy state.

(2) Indirect: Tissues do not absorb the light but react to the chemical signals liberated by the photons. These signals may, for example, stimulate the action of hormones, which are then delivered by the blood to the tissues. The signals that touch off the reaction are the same processes that initiate vision, which is the activation by light of specialized photoreceptor cells. In this case, the eye's photoreceptor cells convert the light energy into a neural signal that is transmitted over the body's neural/endocrine pathways to the area or organ where the indirect effect is seen.

These orthodox explanations constitute the rather limited physical way that current medicine perceives the direct and indirect effects of light, and thus light therapy. In order to understand the powerful effects of The 49th Vibrational Technique and how it actively operates, one must look at not only the physical tissues within the body (direct physical effect) but at the surrounding energy fields that interact with it (indirect physical effect). The human systems themselves (energetic and physical) have constant and incredibly complex interactions that include the mind, emotions and body and their related energies, all of which influence the auric field.

The densest part of the aura closely surrounds the physical body and is known as the health aura (see Diagram 2-1). This energy layer, seen in Tesla-Kirlian photographs, connects the higher energy levels of the aura with the body and allows them to interpenetrate every cell, keeping the body functioning and alive.

As explained in Chapter 2, all diseases, at least in their initial states, are attributable to disturbances in the etheric field or the health aura — that is, at the energy level. Color medicine deals effectively with disease because it treats the body's etheric field. Once the energy balance is restored at etheric levels, it will penetrate into the denser levels of the physical structure within three hours after application. The 49th Vibrational Technique is not a treatment that initially works on the physical body, but it still affects most of the so-called acute, and even chronic, diseases that ail mankind.

In contrast, contemporary medicine utilizes treatments mainly on the physical level, such as surgery or drugs, which often specifically suppress the cleansing symptoms. Destructive results found on life energy can be seen on Tesla-Kirlian photographs. To understand why surgery and drugs often slow (or in some cases prevent) healing, we will give the following simple example: To successfully remove imbalanced energy (the cause of all disease), The 49th Vibrational Technique starts at the higher (etheric) vibrational levels. This is analogous to a mountain stream (live energy) that flows from the mountaintop (the etheric body), gathering particles (toxins) and additional density (tension) as it works its way downstream (to the body). It is obviously simpler to purify the entire river bed by treating it at the time and on the level the pollution first appears (the etheric body) rather than downstream (the physical body). The farther downstream one applies the treatment, the less effective it is. The denser and filthier the stream (or the energy) becomes, the more doubtful the result and the more time-consuming the treatment.

It is interesting to note that the medical profession also uses light therapy or vibrating systems, but they confine themselves to using the infrared and ultraviolet spectra, which can be harmful and are just outside or beyond the beneficial range, visible to the human eye. It is now well known that infrared and ultraviolet rays as well as medically prescribed drugs can be detrimental to health. Newest research, for example, no longer recommends directing infrared lamps toward the head because of possible damage to the higher frequency body area from the low-frequency light. Color medicine, using only the beneficial visible spectrum, especially when combined with a proper dietary routine and avoidance of toxins, is an effective and safe healing method for every home and healing practice in the age of enlightenment.

Eliminating Energy Imbalances

As we have seen, contemporary medicine understands the concept of varying energy levels. However, it focuses on the chemical and physical realm of reaction rather than on the body's etheric energy fields (aura) for providing treatment. While operating with high-frequency rays from the nonbeneficial ranges (like x-rays) or with low-frequency chemical substances, medical treatments may not only suppress the (cleansing) symptoms but also further imbalance the body, as can be proven by Tesla-Kirlian photographs.

To heal the imbalance one of two things is required.

- In the case of an overcharge situation (too-high energy levels), one may utilize the opposite color vibration to neutralize the excess energy in the system. For example, damage from high-energy x-rays or ultraviolet rays (blue end of the spectrum) are counterbalanced by the opposite color, Red.

- In the case of an undercharge situation (too-low energy levels) the balancing color (opposite color) must then be introduced into the etheric body to correct the deficiency. For example, burns from heat (from the red end of the spectrum) are balanced by blue; or underactivity of the liver is balanced by Red, this time in its role as a liver stimulant.

In other words, by adding the appropriate vibrations through The 49th Vibrational Technique, one can heal the physical body through the etheric body, restoring harmony and balance, thus eliminating disease.

The Chemistry of Colors

In the 1920s Dinshah researched the color bands of spectrograms, produced when a chemical element undergoes a process of combustion or vaporization that accelerates the motion of its atoms. The specific bands of colors and dark lines emitted when a certain element is heated are known as Fraunhofer lines. This procedure is now commonly used to identify the chemical composition of a substance (photospectrometry).

Contrary to accepted scientific theory, which assumes that each element is a unit, Dinshah concluded that the chemical elements are actually color compounds. For instance, when he investigated hydrogen, two colors appeared: first a faint blue, and then a very bright, predominant red, together characteristic of that element. Dinshah referred not to an element per se, but always to its predominant color — red in the case of hydrogen, blue for oxygen, yellow for sodium and so on.

From this comes the basis of Dinshah's theory of color healing: the premise that our bodies are made up of chemical elements consisting of a certain balance of color waves or vibrations. A specific disease thus constitutes a specific imbalance of color waves — and, by implication, a

Predominant Color in Spectral Lines of Selected Elements	
Predominant Color	**Spectrogram Emission of Element**
Red:	Hydrogen, Krypton
Orange:	Calcium, Selenium, Copper
Yellow:	Magnesium, Carbon, Sodium
Lemon (the ray richest in minerals):	Germanium, Iron, Gold, Iodine, Silver, Phosphorus, Sulphur, Thorium
Green:	Chlorine, Barium
Turquoise:	Fluorine, Zinc
Blue:	Oxygen, Indium
Indigo	Bismuth, Ionium
Violet:	Cobalt, Actinium
Purple:	Europium, Bromine
Magenta:	Potassium, Lithium

chemical imbalance. Dinshah found that by tonating the body with a particular color vibration one could effectively reintroduce the appropriate biochemical elements into the body. We refer to this as "color chemistry" — certainly a new field of research.

It becomes evident now that color medicine not only can heal the diseased frequencies of the body, but can introduce actual chemical element/vibrations into the body in a nontoxic form.

Reinforcing Chromatherapy with Charged Water and Tissue Salts

As we now understand, color vibrations are carried by light directly into the etheric body and from there to the physical, thereby manifesting even chemical compounds needed in the human body. Since this process ideally requires a one-hour treatment, it may sometimes be more convenient to use an indirect medium as carrier of the healing rays — charged water, for example. This process is called hydrochromatherapy (see Chapter 4). For this purpose water is tonated with the appropriate color and then ingested. The use of hydrochromatherapy can further supplement healing processes by inserting one's dose of the twelve Schuessler tissue salts into charged water. These tissue salts are necessary for our bodies to function properly and are contained in every cell of the body in different concentrations. These tissue salts need to be kept at a balance for vibrant health and vitality, for if one salt is deficient in the body, the others cannot function properly. The proportion of these salts in human tissues corresponds directly to other vital chemical balances on earth and beyond, such as distant stars and planets. Because life came out of the sea, the salt/mineral content of seawater is similar to that of human blood.

As an example, Red- or Orange-charged water, when combined with homeopathic portions of sodium sulphate (nat. sulph.) and iron phosphate (ferr. phos.), respectively, is commonly said to work well on all cold or dormant conditions of the body, as it warms the blood and stimulates the nerves. It is beneficial for deficient menstruation or underfunctioning kidneys. For vibrations from the blue end of the spectrum, calcium sulphate (calc. sulph.) and silicic oxide (silica) are generally recommended, combined with Blue-charged water to slow down the excitable nervous system or brain. Potassium phosphate, when combined with Yellow/Orange-charged water, may function as a laxative, animating the bowels and the nerves. (The twelve tissue salts can be acquired at most full-line health food stores, accompanied by recommendation of dosage.)

Some sources state that a person born with a specific sun sign is lacking a specific tissue salt. Summarized below are the twelve tissue salts (considered deficiency salts) and their corresponding astrological signs (astro-biochemistry), as established by others:

The 12 Tissue Salts & Their Astrological Correlations			
Chemical Compound	Tissue Salt	Common Name	Astrological Sign
K_3HPO_4	Kalium Phosphoricum	Phosphate of potash	Aries
$Na_2SO_4 \cdot 10H_2O$	Natrum Sulphuricum	Sulphate of soda	Taurus
KCl	Kalium Muriaticum	Chloride of potash	Gemini
CaF_2	Calcarea Fluorica	Fluoride of lime	Cancer
$MgHPO_4 \cdot 7H_2O$	Magnesia Phosphorica	Phosphate of magnesia	Leo
K_2SO_4	Kalium Sulphuricum	Sulphate of potash	Virgo
$Na_2HPO_4 \cdot 12H_2O$	Natrum Phosphoricum	Phosphate of soda	Libra
$CaSO_4$	Calcarea Sulphurica	Sulphate of lime	Scorpio
SiO_2	Silica	Silicea	Sagittarius
$Ca_3(PO_4)_2$	Calcarea Phosphorica	Phosphate of lime	Capricorn
NaCl	Natrum Muriaticum	Chloride of soda	Aquarius
$Fe_3(PO_4)_2$	Ferrum Phosphoricum	Phosphate of iron	Pisces

A different research approach called B.E.E.M. has established different relationships. The table on the following page lists its research results, with some correlations still under investigation.

This system does not assume that these correlations necessarily point out deficiency tissue salts, for then every person would be born deficient — that is, diseased.

The Effects of Colored Clothing

Appropriately colored clothing can also play an integral part in the effective absorption of light. Lighter colors reflect the light and darker fabrics absorb it. One would logically think that white clothing, which reflects most of the color rays, would be ineffective for healing. However, part of the white light penetrates the garments and passes into the body. A dark or black garment has an attraction for all rays, preventing their escape and heating up the garment. To a greater or lesser extent the other colors reflect or absorb light and heat, depending on whether they are closer to violet/white or red/black in frequency.

B.E.E.M. Correlation of Tissue Salt, Astrological Sign & Color		
Tissue Salt	**Sun Sign**	**Dinshah Color**
Nat. Mur.	Aries	Magenta
Calc. Sulph.	Taurus	Red
Ferr. Phos.	Gemini	Blue
Calc. Phos.	Cancer	Lemon
Nat. Phos.	Leo	Green
Kali Sulph.	Virgo	Purple
Kali Mur.	Libra	Indigo
Mag. Phos.	Scorpio	Orange
Nat. Sulph.	Sagittarius	Yellow
Calc. Sulph./Nat. Phos./ Kali Phos.	Capricorn	Red, Green, Violet; White
Kali Phos.	Aquarius	Violet
Calc. Fluor.	Pisces	Scarlet
Silica	last 5 days of the year	Turquoise

The fact that the body becomes warmer with dark-colored clothing means that most of the solar energy is absorbed by the garments, thus increasing body heat. White or light-colored clothing has a more uplifting, freeing effect because it permits light to pass into the body and escape from it. Light-colored clothing thus feels cooler.

The color of our clothing also has an effect on the general nature of our skin. For instance, a consistent wearing of black can in time wither the skin. That is, black does not allow sufficient exchange of frequencies; thus the energy gets trapped. When light rays — heat, for example — are completely transmitted into and out of the body, no change in temperature will occur. The exposure to too much light or heat (frequencies), of course, would exhaust the body. This means that the right color vibration, when absorbed by the body, can effect positive changes, be it for necessary sedation via stimulation (black) or stimulation via sedation (white).

To treat a cold, for instance, one wears white clothing for a few days (not the dark, heat-trapping garments we tend to believe appropriate), and quicker recovery results, contrary to expectation. Certain effects also accompany other colors: A garment can, for example, stimulate lungs (orange), liver (red) and kidneys (magenta), as these organs can absorb needed frequencies from our clothing.

Unconsciously choosing the "wrong" color for oneself may mean that the system wants to emphasize the problem to bring it to one's conscious attention for healing. For example, some people with latent kidney problems prefer black, which aggravates the problem. Then they may start preferring magenta or white clothing, which helps to heal the kidneys.

When people are forced to wear certain colors (as in uniforms), discomfort and/or disease may eventually follow. In such cases it is helpful to wear at least a small item of the preferred color on the body to satisfy that need. Environmental colors also influence us, since we absorb color frequencies through the eyes.

How the Color of Foods Affects Us

For purposes of our discussion we will deal with the vibrational, or color, aspect of food rather than its nutritive content. Since foods have their own individual color vibrations, consuming the appropriate foods of the right colors (preferably organically grown and with no additives) can help to balance and rejuvenate the system. Food colors have the same vibrational effect on our bodies as light therapy, but to a lesser degree. Red, orange and yellow foods, for instance, are stimulating. Green foods are neutral, whereas the blue, indigo and violet foods are calming.

Red foods are stimulating: meats, fruits and vegetables with bright red skins such as red apples, tomatoes, peppers.

Orange foods are decongesting: carrots, oranges, tangerines, apricots, peaches.

Yellow foods are uplifting: yellow corn, yellow apples.

Yellow-green (Dinshah Lemon) foods are cleansing: green chili, lemons, limes.

Green foods are balancing: leafy vegetables and fruit with green skin such as olives, peas and cucumbers.

Turquoise plants have healing effects on the skin: aloe vera.

Blue foods are soothing: fish, veal, blue corn.

Indigo foods promote intuition: blueberries.

Violet foods are calming: blue plums.

Purple fruit relaxes: blackberries, purple grapes.

Magenta foods balance the emotions: eggplants, beets.

Scarlet fruits activate: red cherries, strawberries.

The foods we consume are a direct reflection of the forces of nature with its spectral color frequencies, which are responsible for the existence of life and the sustained growth of man, plants and animals. All have a vibrational effect on the cells, tissues, organs and the other interrelated systems (mind, emotions) connected with our bodies.

Other color/food approaches relate to the seven rainbow colors only. Oriental teachings, specifically the Hindu theory of food vibrations, reason that all foods are composed of the seven rays of the cosmos (the rainbow colors) and the five elements (earth, water, fire, air and ether). They state that foods (and their nutritional value) vary in their structure, composition and effectiveness solely by the quantity and quality of the seven rays and the five elements. These teachings further declare that foods have taste only because of the state of disintegration of matter contained within the foods. The preference of taste (or degree of disintegration) obviously varies from culture to culture.

Vibrations of all kinds affect our environment and also directly affect the quality and purity of the food we eat (fertilizers, atmospheric conditions, general pollution, seasonal irregularities, etc.). All apples are *not* created equal. Any polarity imbalance in the environment will affect the quality of foods.

The Vital Elements of Fire, Water and Air in Food

Foods have a polarity — as does everything in the cosmos — characterized by positive, negative and neutral energy. The following are examples of this understanding in connection with these three vital elements.

Electric-Positive Foods (Positive Ions): Hot foods contain the element of fire and are associated with the circulatory system (blood).

Electric-Negative Foods (Negative Ions): Cold foods contain the element of water and are associated with the lymphatic system (lymph).

Electric-Neutral Foods: Foods with the element of air are related to the cerebrospinal system (nerves).

In Ayurvedic thought, any increase or decrease of one or more elements (water, air, fire, ether, earth) in man will affect the interrelated but somewhat independent systems of the body, thus determining ones needs and character. Therefore, there are different types of people with different element/food/vibration needs, classified in Ayurvedic medicine as air-ether, fire-water and water-earth personalities.

Air-ether personalities *(vata)* are slender, with a light bone structure. They are philosophers and love to travel, but often have weak nerves, pains and digestive problems. For them, foods of the calming blue/green type like asparagus, olives, green beans, blueberries or avocado are recommended.

Fire-water personalities *(pitta)* have a strong bone structure and are moderate in weight. They are intelligent, energetic and generally like to lead. They have allergies and suffer from headaches and acidity. For them, cleansing foods like cool salads, fruits, juices and liquids are recommended, with frequencies around green (lemon, green, turquoise). They may eat heavy meals two or three times a day, for they digest food easily.

Water-earth personalities *(kapha)* are often overweight with a heavy bone structure. They like business and are money-oriented. They may suffer circulatory and heart diseases. They enjoy stimulating foods like cakes, sweets, grains, beans and vegetables. It is mainly the carbohydrate, red type of food that is recommended and is not too fattening when consumed in its natural state (whole grains and natural sugars). Water-earth people love to eat and their bodies seem to demand more and more.

By ancient tradition the Indian Ayurvedic science of health recommends only vegetarian foods to balance polarity (vibrations). This is extremely important in keeping the acid-alkaline balance in the blood and checking disease (blocked energy). Changes from a meat to a health diet should, however, as a rule, be done gradually, except in emergencies.

How Polarity and Foods Interrelate

There are other theories about food vibrations that are also classified by polarity, such as electric negative/electric positive; *yin/yang*;
feminine/masculine equivalents. The *yin* is the feminine, electric negative ion, or blue, indigo, purple, green and white foods; the *yang* is the
masculine, electric positive ion, or red, orange, brown and black foods.
Locations or climates on the planet where foods should be consumed for
the best polarity or affinity should also be recognized. For instance, in
hot countries rice is recommended, as it contains predominantly the
water element; in cold countries wheat is preferred, as it contains the fire
element.

The process of metabolism in humans (described earlier) is in some
respects a reversal of the process of plant synthesis. Plants draw on light
(color), and through the process of photosynthesis the plant grows. Man
consumes the plant (light/color), which is then absorbed into the body to
replenish the colors of the aura; the aura in turn emits light.

The process comes full circle, and any deviation from the normal
cosmic vibrations — too little or too much light/color and other frequencies — in the food we consume may produce energy inappropriate for the
human body, especially for an already diseased system.

A full discourse on the effects and vibratory/element rate for food is
a subject for other publications. We must, however, note that contemporary nutrition has overlooked the value of balancing the
vibratory/color rate of food within the body.

Astrological or Cosmic Color Rays

Astrological charts indicate that man's activity during his life span is
influenced to some degree by the cosmic forces and especially by the
major planetary aspects or relationships at the time of birth. This can be
understood by the vibrations (frequencies) that the planets emit in-
dividually and in combination. Many of these vibrations, of course,
strike the earth and some can be measured.

Various sources relate the sun signs to color vibrations. Below is a list of colors that, as some sources say, individuals may *lack* astrological-ly, inasmuch as the vibrations (colors) were lacking at the time of their birth due to the specific alignment of the planets. These assertions are given here as information only and need to be verified by further research.

Sun-Sign Color Deficiencies	
Aquarius	blue, white rays
Pisces	green, white rays
Aries	red rays
Taurus	yellow rays
Gemini	yellow and purple rays
Cancer	white and green rays
Leo	orange and yellow rays
Virgo	violet and gold rays
Libra	crimson and gold rays
Scorpio	red and scarlet rays
Sagittarius	red and green rays
Capricorn	green rays

If the assumptions are correct, these deficiency colors should be incorporated into one's diet or clothing on a regular or frequent basis. Another approach (see below) shows different sun sign/color correlations based on the ancient wisdom, reintroduced and developed in the B.E.E.M system.

B.E.E.M. Sun-Sign/Color Correlations			
Aquarius	Violet	Leo	Green
Pisces	Scarlet	Virgo	Purple
Aries	Magenta	Libra	Indigo
Taurus	Red	Scorpio	Orange
Gemini	Blue	Sagittarius	Yellow
Cancer	Lemon	Capricorn	White

These colors are to be understood as vibrationally related to the sun signs. Some of the color/sign correlations of this system are still being researched.

Why can we assume that a relationship between sun signs (the earth-related zodiacal position of the sun) and colors exists? Because all cosmic entities (planets, man, animals, plants, etc.) are directly influenced by cosmic vibrations — and in turn influence the cosmos. The cycles and relative positions of the heavenly bodies influence the growing seasons, hemispheric location, time of the year, weather patterns, temperature, etc. This influence is scientifically recognized, since the position of the planets determines the angle and intensity of their rays, which affect life on earth.

The different angles that a planet's energy strikes the earth has an effect similar to that of the different angles at which the sun's rays strike at various seasons and times of day. It not only affects the growing cycle, but also the soil, its mineral and vitamin content, the growth rate and the vibrations of the foods we consume.

We can see how the position of the moon affects our tides, our emotional and physical body functions and how the rhythm of the universe repeats itself annually with the four seasons. All these recognizable changes confirm that energy (light/color) has an influence on humans, who are born within this cosmic energy envelope to grow and eventually die within it.

4

Color Practice

Materials and Practical Techniques for Applying Color Medicine

The Twelve Color Filters and Light Sources

THE FILTERS. The plastic color transparencies (filters or gels) that are used in The 49th Vibrational Technique can be obtained from reliable sources and are quite simple to use. It is important to note that these twelve colors are correlated with scientific precision and cannot be replaced by a hue of the same color name. Each color must be a derivative of the same harmonious primary vibration in order to have the correct combination of colors tuned to the aura for healing. The early treatments of color therapy used glass filters. However, they had to be precisely tuned to each other in an expensive process and were easily broken and difficult to replace. The one disadvantage to plastic filters is that they can melt under extreme heat without the protection of a heat shield. Treated properly, they may last indefinitely. Also, the heat shield should not get too close to the light source nor heated beyond a certain point.

One can make the filters from sheets of exact colors available in inexpensive, high-quality plastic material. The best, most reliable heat-resistant color sheets are the Roscolux products manufactured by the

Rosco Laboratories, 36 Bush Avenue, Port Chester, New York 10573, USA (914) 937-1300. Rosco has a worldwide network of dealers who offer these plastic sheets carefully numbered by color. In most metropolitan areas distributors can be located in the Yellow Pages under Theatrical Supplies.

To make the color filters, one needs to acquire ten of the different Roscolux 20x24-inch sheets to be able to make (cut) the twelve appropriate color filters for The 49th Vibrational Technique system. These are numbered: 15, 24, 25, 47, 59, 69, 79, 86A, 90 and 389. The corresponding colors and numbers (nine of them need to be assembled) are as follows:

Commercial Filter Combinations for Precise Frequencies	
49th-Vibration Color	Roscolux Filter #
Red	818, 828
Orange	809, 828
Yellow	809
Lemon	809, 871
Green	871
Turquoise	861, 871
Blue	859, 866
Indigo	828, 859, 866
Violet	832, 859, 866
Purple	832, 866
Magenta	818, 828, 866
Scarlet	810, 818, 861

In putting the different sheets together to make a specific color filter, the order of colors does not matter. The sheets are cut to the appropriate size and affixed together by staples or clear tape.

THE HEAT SHIELD. This should be purchased with the color sheets and placed between the light source and the filters for maximum filter life. This is important when using higher-wattage bulbs or when the light source is relatively close to the filter. A heat shield is mandatory when using a quartz lamp, because it eliminates the ultraviolet rays found in this type of lamp.

THE FILTER HOLDER. Metal inserts (filter holders) can be obtained from the same source as the sheets and affixed to the front of the lamp, where the filters can be inserted. Heat-resistant tape or wire will hold the metal insert best. An inexpensive filter holder can also be made of a folded piece of cardboard. Holes must be cut in the center of both sides to let the light pass through (Diagram 4-1).

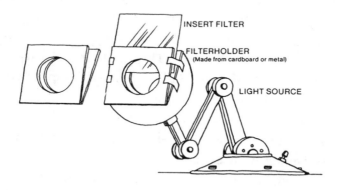

INSERT FILTER

FILTERHOLDER
(Made from cardboard or metal)

LIGHT SOURCE

Diagram 4-1. Filter holder and light source. Transformation of any regular household light into therapy light. Any incandescent light source can be used. The filter holder may be constructed from cardboard or metal and taped to light source. If heat shield is used, insert behind filter on the bulb side.

THE LIGHT SOURCE. Any incandescent lamp with a single opening for the light can serve as a source for The 49th Vibrational Technique to tonate (shine) the colored light on the body (a desk lamp, reading light, etc.). Since the kilowatt power is not of major importance, a 25-, 60- or 100-watt bulb will be quite sufficient to apply (radiate) the color vibrations effectively. There is often a misconception that the higher the wattage, the more effective the results. As in sound therapy, it is not the volume (wattage) but the pitch (exact color frequency) that counts. A 100-watt bulb enclosed in a housing placed on a stand is sufficient for even professional use. These devices can be purchased in theatrical supply stores or through the most comprehensive supplier of theatrical lighting: Times Square Lighting, 318 W. 47th Street, NYC, New York 10036, (212) 245-4155.

Some practitioners of color therapy utilize 300- to 1000-watt incandescent bulbs, which can be beneficial in some cases. However, a 60- or 100-watt bulb, when used for the recommended one hour, will generally be equally effective and has a longer and thus more cost-efficient life. Larger-wattage bulbs may be desired for visual purposes in meditation or in some chronic conditions. Other chronic conditions may respond better to extremely low wattage (15 watts or less). Quartz bulbs are very effective, as they have the whitest light; however, they definitely require the use of heat shields to filter out their ultraviolet rays, which could eventually damage even closed eyes. The possibility of harmful side effects from extensive use of quartz bulbs when used with a heat shield has not yet been established.

Some of the most successful tonations can be accomplished in direct sunlight by taking one or more 20 x 24-inch Roscolux sheets to make a large filter, suspending it on a frame over the appropriate part of the body. The filters should not touch the skin, to avoid discomfort caused by heavy perspiration. A heat shield is definitely required.

Needless to say, fluorescent tubes are not suitable for color therapy, as they contain mercury or lead and operate at an interfering frequency. Once the colored light source is established, the room then needs to be carefully prepared for the tonation.

Preparations

THE ROOM. All toxins must be removed from the air space of the room and of the environment for healing to be effective. An ideal situation is to be in a quiet, totally dark room at 80 degrees F (28 degrees C), although total darkness is not necessary. The lack of any other type of light rays will render more effective the specific colors emanating from the tonation source. The temperature level is extremely important, since it relaxes the physical body, thus allowing more light to be absorbed by the aura. If the room is too cool, the body will be tensed or give up some of its energy to combat the cold at the expense of absorbing the healing rays. An electric heater may be used to warm the body if necessary.

PREPARING THE BODY. For best results one should not eat or bathe at least one hour before or after a tonation in order to let the aura settle. No tonation should be given during menstruation except when excessive bleeding or pain is present, because at that time the body is already cleansing and balancing itself. The body's heart and respiratory rates should be checked to see if the ratio is in the most beneficial 5:1 range (discussed later in this chapter). The tonation is applied for one hour on the bare skin (the area of the health aura). A shorter duration is less effective. The light is directed onto the appropriate body area (Affected Area — AA) as outlined in Chapter 5, on the systemic front or back (SF, SB) or on the whole-body front or back (WBF, WBB).

The individual must be as relaxed as possible for optimal absorption of the colored rays by the aura. The eyes may be closed or open, at the individual's option. One can meditate, relax or sleep. Sleeping babies should have their eyes covered when being tonated to ensure sound rest.

Body Orientation and Absorption Time

SUPINE POSITION. The 49th Vibrational Technique is most effective when the individual lies on his or her back or side with the crown of the head toward magnetic north. Lying parallel to the earth's magnetic field aligns the body and its electrical polarities (the liver and the spleen). Lying on one's stomach when utilizing The 49th Vibrational Technique is not advisable, as that position is said to reverse the body's electrical poles in relation to the earth. When one is tonating the back of the body, one needs to be lying on one's side, with the crown of the head pointing toward magnetic north. Lying down is preferred, as the circulatory system is under the least stress with this orientation (Diagram 4-2).

Distractions, such as radio or television, are not recommended, because during the tonating process (except for the twelve suggested monochord 49th Vibrational Technique healing tapes or other healing tapes) it is important that the body's electromagnetic field or aura not be disturbed by interfering frequencies.

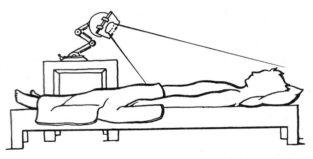

Diagram 4-2. Treatment unit, supine position for systemic front.
Crown of head points north, chest and head elevated by pillow to
avoid shadows on upper chest. Bare the skin for systemic front (SF)
from hip joints to above the head. Room is darkened and heated to
80° F (28° C); electric heater may be used to warm the body. Any
incandescent light source can be used with any available wattage.
However, the exact color filters are essential. Tonation time: one
hour.

SITTING POSITION. If for any reason it is undesirable to lie
down for the color treatment, an alternative approach is to sit facing
south during the treatment (back of head toward north), to keep the
body's polarity in alignment with the earth's magnetic field (Diagram
4-3).

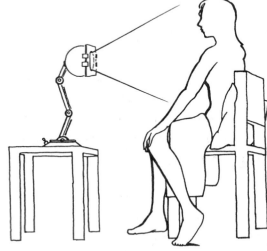

Diagram 4-3. Treatment unit, sitting position for systemic front.
Back of head is to north. Room, light, filters etc. analogous to
Diagram 4-2.

BRIGHTNESS AND FREQUENCY. When using The 49th Vibrational Technique keep in mind that all colors do not necessarily appear with the same intensity (brightness, luminosity). However, the healing effect on the aura is not dependent on luminosity, but on the proper frequencies; the brightness is secondary for the aura to receive the energy or vibrations. What is essential, however, is that filters be of the correct frequency and the light be applied to the bare skin.

SUMMARY. One needs (1) a light source with a 25- to 100-watt incandescent light bulb (or quartz lamp with heat shield); (2) a room temperature of 80 degrees F (or electric space heater to warm the body); (3) relative darkness, concentrating the light source through the filter onto the bare skin of the appropriate part of the body (as outlined in Chapter 5); (4) the lamp to be a meter (or yard) or more above and behind the feet or, alternatively, above or beside the body, with crown of head toward north in supine position; and (5) tonation time ideally one hour.

Using More Than One Color in a Session

When using two different colors at the same time (no more than two in one session), one must use either two of the warm colors (Red, Orange, Yellow, Lemon or Green) or two of the cool colors (Green, Turquoise, Blue, Indigo or Violet). Since Green is neutral, it can be considered either warm or cool. Purple can be used with Magenta, as can Magenta with Scarlet. When using two colors simultaneously, it is important that the rays not overlap and that the eyes remain closed, thus avoiding a blending of the colors either in the eyes or on the body surface so that one color does not dominate the other or produce altered frequencies.

Selecting the Areas and the Timing

TONATION AREAS OF THE BODY. The twelve healing colors or vibrations inherent in The 49th Vibrational Technique are Red, Orange, Yellow, Lemon, Green, Turquoise, Blue, Indigo, Violet, Purple, Magenta and Scarlet. They can be selected from color schedules (Chapter 5).

A single color or several colors as given in the color schedules are generally applied to the body one after the other, session by session, on the appropriate area(s) (see Diagram 5-1 in Chapter 5). Color medicine is often most beneficial when the tonations are applied to the "systemic front" (from hip joints to top of head, front side) or "systemic back" (from hip joints to top of head, back side) (see Diagram 5-1). Colored light is fully effective only when applied to the front or back of the body or to appropriate organ areas without the interference of clothing.

TONATION SEQUENCE. It takes approximately one to three hours after a treatment for the color vibrations that are placed on the aura to be totally absorbed into the physical body. It is definitely not recommended that tonations be done consecutively hour by hour. For this reason, when using The 49th Vibrational Technique, one should wait at least one hour (two is preferred) after one tonation before starting a second one. EXCEPTION: Turquoise or Green can be used for lengthy tonations, if required. Green is effective for oncoming colds and Turquoise works well for healing burns and wounds after Blue or Indigo. This rule to wait at least one hour between tonations must of course be waived when an emergency requires immediate change in color or constant attention. If a continuous tonation is given that exceeds the one-hour period (in general, not to be done with colors other than Turquoise or Green), it is imperative that the person taking the tonation not look into the direct light. If one is on a fairly moderate program of tonations in general (one a day), the eyes can remain open. In many cases it is beneficial for the light to penetrate the eyes. However, the body itself will tell which is most comfortable, eyes open or closed. It is generally important to follow this lead.

OPTIMIZED TONATION TIME. There is no fixed time of day for a color tonation to be most effective. However, one's openness for the treatment can be an important factor. In general, the stimulating colors (Red, Orange, Yellow, Lemon and Scarlet) are the most effective for daytime use. The sedating or neutral colors (Turquoise, Blue, Indigo, Violet, Magenta and Green) are more for the late afternoon or evenings.

Although The 49th Vibrational Technique has been reported to be effective when used for less than an hour even in daylight, maximum results are more likely when one follows the recommendations.

Interaction of Heart and Respiratory Rates (Dinshah Ratio)

THE HEALTH RATIO. In color medicine one needs to understand the interrelationship between the body's heart and respiratory rates as researched by Dinshah. In order for color therapy to be most effective, these two rates (or their ratio) need to be in proper balance for the energy within the body to function optimally. A ratio of 5:1 is considered ideal (the heart rate being the higher and the respiration rate being the lower), although 4:1 or 6:1 is still sufficient for healing purposes. For the heart rate, the pulse is taken with a finger (not the thumb) at the wrist on the thumb's side of the middle ligament for one minute. In calculating the respiration rate we deal with a complete breathing cycle (one inhalation and one exhalation equals one cycle). For instance, if the heart rate is 75 beats per minute (considered about normal, higher in children) and the respiratory rate is 15 cycles per minute, that ratio is 5:1 — that is, 75 divided by 15. Or:

$$\frac{\text{Heartbeat (pulse/min.)}}{\text{Respiration (a complete breath)}} = \frac{75}{15} = \frac{5}{1} = 5 \text{ Dinshah Health Ratio}$$

RESPIRATORY RATE TOO HIGH (RATIO <5). When the heartbeat is about normal but breathing is too rapid (for example, 75 beats per minute and 25 cycles per minute = 75:25, or 3:1), the lungs have to work excessively to receive the appropriate amount of oxygen (Blue), and often do not properly release carbon dioxide and toxins. One then needs to relax the respiratory system with Indigo, tonated on the lung area (back or front), to make respiration more effective.

RESPIRATORY RATE TOO LOW (RATIO >5). When the heart rate is about normal and breathing too slow (for example, 75 beats per minute and 10 cycles per minute = 75:10, or 7.5:1), the body is not getting enough oxygen because the lungs are fatigued, or perhaps because the breathing center in the brain is damaged by toxins and thus unable to help detoxify the body. Here the lungs need to be activated with Orange, tonated on the lung area (back or front) in sequence with a general detoxification of environment and body (mainly by using Lemon on the body).

HEART RATE. A normal heart rate for adults lies between 55 beats per minute (found mainly in athletes and vegetarians) and 85 beats per minute (nonvegetarians), obviously depending on one's diet, physical exercise, lifestyle, and gender. Should the heart rate be higher or lower than normal and the respiratory rate near normal, one then needs to adjust the heart rate to balance the ratio.

HEART RATE TOO HIGH (RATIO >5). With too fast a heartbeat and a normal breathing rate (for example, 105 beats per minute and 15 cycles per minute = 105/15, or 7:1), the heart needs to be calmed by Purple tonated on the heart area (front).

HEART RATE TOO LOW (RATIO <5). With too slow a heartbeat and a normal breathing rate (for example, 45 beats per minute and 15 cycles per minute = 45/15, or 3:1), the heart needs to be stimulated by Scarlet tonated on the heart area (front).

CHECKING HEART RATE. If one is unsure whether the heart rate is too high or too low for a specific individual — since this can change due to age, exercise and nutrition — one should note the ratio. Tonate then with Magenta for one hour or for a few sessions on upper chest (front) and/or kidney area (back), and take the ratio again. If the heart rate has become higher, this indicates that it needs to be higher, so one tonates with Scarlet in the next session. If the heart rate becomes lower after Magenta, then it needs to be lower, and one follows with Purple.

RATIO SUMMARY:

Ratio 5:1	Good health or good chance for recovery.
Ratio 4:1	Relatively good health and relatively good chance for recovery.
Ratio 3:1	Urgent care needed, possibly toxic.
Ratio 2:1 (or lower)	Death may be near, yet recovery is always possible

Ratio 6:1 (or higher) Toxins may be taxing the heart or the respir-ation center
(as found by B.E.E.M. research) in the brain. Body is possibly affected by toxicity.

IMPORTANCE OF THE RATIO. Before getting actively involved in the application of The 49th Vibrational Technique, one needs to calculate this ratio to determine if one's heart rate and respiratory cycles are functioning correctly and therefore more responsive to treatment. It is important that these two life-energy systems function in the 4:1, 5:1 or 6:1 range.

In severe cases the treatment of major symptoms should begin immediately. In instances that are not critical, one should fine-tune the heart/lung ratio to a healthy range before commencing treatment.

DETERIORATION OF RATIO ADJUSTMENT. When the ratio falls back into imbalance within a few days after a color medicine adjustment, this may indicate a toxic environment. Look for toxins polluting the air (pesticides, mothballs, herbicides, laundry products, tobacco smoke etc.) in or around the environment and remove or neutralize them.

Hydrochromatherapy: Color-Charged Water as a Healing Supplement

INTERNAL COLOR THERAPY. Vibrational therapy can also be practiced through the use of charged water (hydrochromatherapy). This can serve a dual purpose: receiving color and additional water, as most people do not consume enough water daily. One can devise a system where a color filter can be set atop a container of water, using either direct sunlight (most effective) or an incandescent light to charge the water with the appropriate healing vibrations.

WATER AND CONTAINER. When adding vibrations to the water (charging), it is important to make sure that the liquid itself is pure and receives only the specific colored light rays. One way is to place the water in a glass container and seal it in a dark structure — for example, a black plastic bag used for photo paper or a dark box with its only opening at the top of the glass container where the light filter is placed.

LIGHT SOURCES FOR HYDROCHROMATHERAPY. It has been said that Yellow, Orange, and Red work well when charged with incandescent light, which is on the red/yellow side of the spectrum. The other colors are more effectively charged by natural sunlight, which contains all color rays in a perfect blend. However, the use of both sources has proven to be beneficial in color medicine.

By leaving the container in direct sunlight for a period of three to four hours, the water will be fully charged and ready for consumption. The water should be consumed not long thereafter, as it loses its charge with time. The full range of the twelve colors can be utilized.

STORING CHARGED WATER. When the filter, glass and charged water are removed from the light, it is appropriate to keep the water cool and in a dark place or dark container if it is not to be consumed immediately.

CHARGING WATER DURING TONATION. Many prepare charged water during the color-therapy treatment described earlier. When this is desired, a clear glass filled with water can be placed in the colored light near the person receiving the tonation. The water, taking on color vibration, supplements the aura tonation when subsequently consumed. The artificial light source (*never* use fluorescent light) should be within a yard/meter of the water glass. The liquid should be charged with only one color at a time and then consumed.

ADVANTAGES OF CHARGED WATER. Charged water is a time-saving supplement and most effective when the water directly interacts with the organs or affected areas, such as an ulcer in the digestive or eliminative tracts, where Lemon or Indigo can be beneficial. Yellow-charged water once, then Indigo-charged water can be taken for diarrhea. Lemon, Yellow and Orange are used to overcome constipation. Yellow acts as a laxative, Lemon detoxifies, and Orange activates potassium for acid/alkaline balance. Indigo calms nerves and digestion. When ingesting charged water, the color vibrations also reach many additional areas of the body.

Other situations — such as cleansing the bladder or urinary tract, removing kidney stones, dealing with alcoholism, drug problems and food poisoning, to mention only a few — can be positively affected with hydrochromatherapy along with colored light therapy (see schedules, Chapter 5, for appropriate colors). Charged water can also be quite effective for sound sleep, as consuming Blue-charged water prior to retiring can sooth and relax the stomach.

TONATION OR INGESTION. The use of charged water is most effective when diseases are not chronic or acute. Acute or chronic situations respond much better to the direct application of light on the aura, using hydrochromatherapy as a supplement to the light treatment. Hydrochromatherapy has the ability to keep the body fine-tuned when applied on a regular and constant basis, assisting in the long- or short-term needs of the aura.

PURIFYING WATER. If one is concerned about the source of one's drinking water (in terms of additives such as toxic fluorides and other industrial contaminants), one can also enhance the water by placing a Lemon filter over the water in a dark container. However, purified bottled water or spring water is recommended for hydrochromatherapy in the absence of a proper water-purification system. The long-term use of distilled water for drinking purposes may deplete the system of vital minerals.

COLOR APOTHECARY. The assortment of the twelve filters of The 49th Vibrational Technique can function as a mini drug store, pulling from the skies the "celestial medicine" that effectively operates our system. Once the body's energy resumes its balance (in terms of vibrations) with chromatherapy and hydrochromatherapy, the system should remain well balanced through daily use of charged water alone unless emotional or environmental toxins massively interfere.

Sound/Light Vibrations for Healing

CONVERTING FROM LIGHT TO SOUND. Color therapy can be effectively supplemented by the use of harmonious sound frequencies. Dinshah calculated the equivalent sound vibration for each of his twelve colors (see Diagram 4-4). For instance, the basic frequency or vibration of the color Red is 436 trillion cycles per second. To arrive at a comparable vibration in the audible range (reducing the vibrations from visual to audible), Dinshah divided the basic color frequency by two, 40 times. That results in 392 for Red, or the musical note G. Through this calculation we find that the corresponding sound is in the range of the ninth theoretical octave — that is, 40 theoretical octaves below the color vibration of the visible spectrum.

THE OCTAVE OF SIX. In music an octave (meaning eight) shares its first and last tones (among its eight notes) with the previous (lower) and following (higher) octaves, respectively. Thus it can be said to consist of seven notes of its own. Interestingly, Dinshah mathematically arrived at only six whole-step notes (G, A, B, C, D, E) as approximate equivalents of the visible 49th octave for Red, Orange, Lemon, Green, Blue and Violet. That is, the previous or following notes would fall, when compared with harmonious light vibrations, in the infrared or ultraviolet ranges. Dinshah added three half-step notes between G and E (A#, C# and D#) for Yellow, Turquoise and Indigo. He combined G and E (that is, Red and Violet) to find the sound equivalent for Magenta; combined A# and E (Yellow and Violet) for Purple; but used G# and D (instead of G and D for Red and Blue) for Scarlet, due to his color/sound correlations.

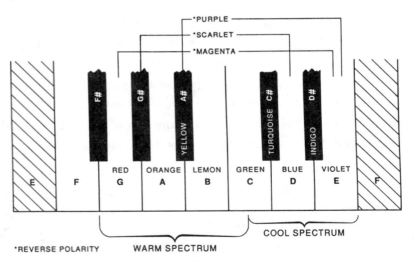

Diagram 4-4. Dinshah color-sound equivalents. Tonal piano complements of color vibrations utilized by The 49th Vibrational Technique. Lower frequencies stimulate; slower rhythms sedate. Purple, Scarlet and Magenta have reversed polarity.

HOW MUSICAL SOUNDS HEAL. Since color, or vibrational therapy, works on the aura, the equivalent color frequencies (notes) also resonate musically in harmony with the color frequencies in the energy field. Utilizing Dinshah's reduction formula, the lower end of the 49th octave, red, equals 392 (decimals omitted) or the note G. This vibration falls in mid-range of most musical instruments, as do the other eleven colors/notes used in color medicine. (See Diagram 4-5 for color/note equivalents.)

It may have been noted that in The 49th Vibrational Technique reds are related to lower sound frequencies (lower in pitch) and blues are related to the higher frequencies (higher pitch) because the vibrations (and therefore the corresponding sounds) of the blues are higher and the reds lower when reduced systematically by Dinshah's formula from color vibrations. Yet keep in mind that for presently unknown reasons, slow rhythms relax (like the blues) and fast rhythms stimulate (like the reds).

The sound/light correlations preferred in The 49th Vibrational Technique for healing are different from those used for purposes of musical entertainment. When matched with discotheque lights, the blues are related to sounds of lower frequencies (lower in pitch); reds are thought to match with sounds of higher frequencies (higher in pitch).

Because it is the matched vibration that heals by its effects through the human aura, harmonious sounds reinforce colored-light therapy tremendously.

USING A SYNTHESIZER FOR ENHANCED COLOR HEALING. Musical instruments that can produce a continuous note, such as a synthesizer, are capable of producing precise frequencies that are harmonious with those of the visible light spectrum when using Dinshah's mathematical formula. Sound, used in tandem with light therapy, multiplies the benefits. Sound alone is, as a rule, not nearly as effective as color medicine, but working synergistically, they are even more powerful. A synthesizer has the ability to intermix many diverse instruments, all tuned to the same vibrational level to make the sound more interesting.

COLOR/SOUND EQUIVALENTS. The equivalent sounds for colors suggested in The 49th Vibrational Technique, as researched by

Dinshah, are summarized on the facing page.

Audio cassette tapes (each tape fixed on a set musical color/ note or vibration of The 49th Vibrational Technique) are available. The six tapes are designed to supplement the twelve colors in the visible spectrum and contain the twelve musical notes or frequencies. Each tape is 30 minutes long. The tapes utilize a synthesizer, with alternating sounds keyed into the specific monochord reduction formula for color therapy and chakra enhancement.

Color Medicine for Animals and Plants

An interesting sideline to color medicine relates to pets and other animals, even though their anatomy is somewhat different from ours. They do, however, have the same basic cellular activity, so that light therapy will accomplish many of the same results within their bodies. Needless to say, we have a difficult or different situation in terms of determining diseases within animals. However, arthritic problems, for instance, can be rectified or reversed in animals as well as in humans utilizing the same color scheme. A pendulum can also be used to determine the appropriate color for animals and plants. It should be noted that animals are often more sensitive and receptive to color medicine than people and thus may need shorter sessions.

The following (and last) chapter deals with the specific application of The 49th Vibrational Technique to more than 100 of mankind's most common diseases. This chapter matches the colors or vibrations with the energy blockages in specific parts of the body.

5

Color Schedule Application

Determining the Appropriate Color(s) for
Relieving/Healing the Major 123 Illnesses

The Treatment of Specific Diseases with Color Medicine

COLOR SCHEDULES. At the end of this chapter (Appendix) there is an alphabetized list of over one hundred of the most common diseases. This list is cross-referenced with the appropriate color filters that should be applied on the various parts of the body to effect the healing process, utilizing The 49th Vibrational Technique.

These color applications for relief and balance follow the Dinshah School, and the necessary colors for the (alphabetized) diseases given in the list are recommended for typical situations. However, some variation might be necessary — even the use of opposite colors, since each individual situation can vary, as can the causes of identical symptoms. In general, the listed colors should be rotated systematically to be totally effective, especially in chronic or acute cases. When there is some doubt about the effects of the colors, rotate one by one until the results can be judged; then concentrate mainly on the color that appears to be most effective at that time. After extended periods of tonations with one color, in order to offer counterbalance to the body, the use of one of the opposite colors is appropriate, as explained in earlier chapters — mainly once in every seven sessions.

Matching the Color Vibrations to the Various Parts of the Body

BODY CHART. A body chart (Diagram 5-1), is given for application of The 49th Vibrational Technique on specifically affected areas (AA). This indicates by number (referred to in the color schedules) the appropriate organ areas of the human body. Diagram 5-2 depicts the

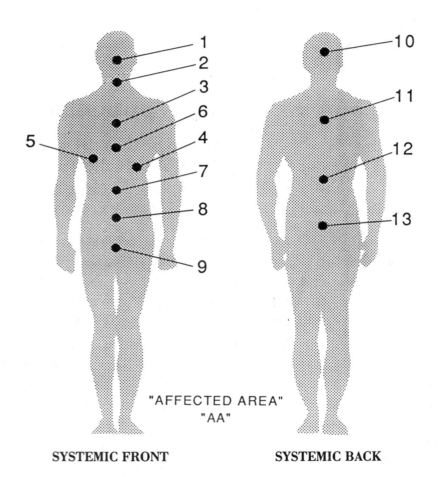

"AFFECTED AREA"
"AA"

SYSTEMIC FRONT   SYSTEMIC BACK

Diagram 5-1. Tonation areas. Left: systemic front (SF, 1–9); right: systemic back (SB, 10–13). The code numbers (shown above) found in the schedules in the Appendix refer to areas where specific organs are found. The main organs within each body area are shown in Diagram 5-2

major organs of the body by specific location. Areas given in the color schedules may also be coded SF, SB, AA, WBF or WBB, indicating whether tonations will need to cover systemic front (SF), systemic back (SB), specifically affected areas (AA), or the whole-body front (WBF) or whole-body back (WBB).

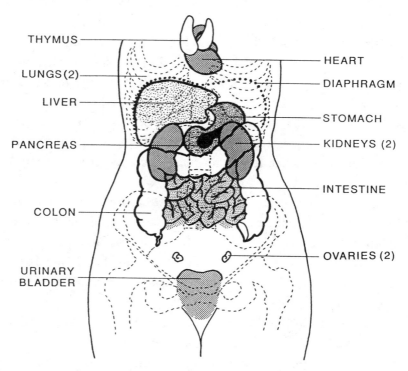

Diagram 5-2. Locations of the major organs.

SYSTEMIC FRONT (SF). Systemic front (Diagram 5-1) covers the area of the seven major chakras and starts with the top of the head, ending at the hip joints (numbers 1-9); on bare skin. Much of the healing process of color therapy relates to utilizing the various colors on this body area. The designated concept will be SF, which means systemic front.

SYSTEMIC BACK (SB). Systemic back (numbers 10-13, shown in Diagram 5-1; bare skin) relates to the back body section, from top of the head down to the hip joints where the major chakras are rooted, designated for tonation purposes as SB (systemic back). Tonation used in The 49th Vibrational Technique needs to specifically cover this entire general area, when so specified.

WHOLE BODY, FRONT OR BACK (WBF, WBB). Whole-body front (WBF) or whole-body back (WBB) includes arms and legs with systemic front or back areas (on bare skin). This is sometimes necessary, for example, in certain blood or skin disorders.

SPECIFICALLY AFFECTED AREAS (AA). When specific areas for improvement are involved (not utilizing the SF or SB), they are designated as (AA), or affected area(s). For reinforcement of these areas, tonation does not require covering the entire front or back chakra areas with colored light. Untreated areas may be covered by clothing, a blanket or similar covering. A number will be designated and coordinated with the specific tonation area, which can then be cross-referenced to Diagram 5-1.

In Diagram 5-1, on the frontal side, we have Area 1, the pituitary, pineal and brain region; Area 2, the neck, thyroid and parathyroid; Area 3, the lungs, heart and thymus; Area 4, the spleen; Area 5, the liver/gall bladder; Area 6, the stomach; Area 7, the small and large intestines; Area 8, the bladder, appendix and internal reproductive organs; and Area 9, the external reproductive organs.

On the back side, Diagram 5-1, are Area 10, the brain; Area 11, the lungs; Area 12, the kidneys; Area 13, the rectum.

When one centers the light ray on the appropriate spot on the body, this will tonate a larger area than shown on the chart, which is the proper organ area.

How to Use the Color Schedules

Looking up "concussion" in the color schedule, for example, one reads: "Purple on SF, Indigo on 1." This means that in the case of concussion one tonates the body systemic front (SF, from hip joints to above head) with the color Purple for one hour. Waiting at least one hour thereafter, one tonates Indigo on the face (Area 1 as seen in Diagram 5-1). The intermediate hour may have to be waived in emergencies. If further relief is necessary, one rotates the colors and tonates with Purple again (SF, systemic front), followed by Indigo on the face (Area 1), etc. Medical examination may be needed first.

Focusing the Colors on the Body

When applying the colors to the body, the lighter shades will be more visible than the darker ones. In the case of some of the darker colors such as Magenta, it becomes more difficult to focus the light on the precise area, especially when that area is important. If one has problems adjusting the darker colors to fit the appropriate area, one can initially insert a lighter-color filter to determine how much of the body is being covered, and then substitute the darker color appropriate for the treatment. The fact that these darker colors are not as visible does not mean that they are not working as effectively as the brighter ones. It is not the brightness of the color but the correct frequency that is crucial.

Checking the Ratio First

Before the first tonation take the ratio and, if time permits, start with the appropriate color to balance the ratio (see Chapter 4). It may be essential to get the respiration/heart-rate ratio in the 5:1 range. If over an extended period of time one has difficulty raising or keeping the ratio above 3:1, for instance, this is a sign that the 49th Vibrational Technique will be very difficult to apply with positive results to the specific person. In this case one may also think of toxins in the environment of, or in use by, this person (air, water, food, and clothing). The toxins have to be removed in order to regain health. If the ratio is in the area of 2:1, it indicates that the person may have very little time left on this planet, yet recovery has been made even then.

Ending a Tonation Cycle

When the system has been cleansed of the energy blockage or disease through The 49th Vibrational Technique, it is then important to take a final tonation with a color in the center of the spectrum (usually Green or Turquoise) to obtain a stabilizing effect.

When the Colors Do Not Work

A DIFFERENT COLOR MAY BE NEEDED. Although The 49th Vibrational Technique has worked rapidly for many, some individuals initially become discouraged while using color medicine when the results are not instantaneous. Many variables enter the picture. At one point a different color might be needed, which the body itself will tell you over a period of several treatments by subsequent comfort and relief.

SUPPORT THROUGH DIET. In many instances, color medicine needs to be used in combination with an appropriate diet, especially in chronic or acute cases where the balance of the auric energy must be coordinated with that of the internal organs.

REMOVING ALL TOXINS. All toxins need to be removed from the working and living areas for healing to take place. This is essential.

AVOIDING UNFAVORABLE REACTIONS. Generally, unfavorable reactions rarely occur, since the aura normally will not absorb unneeded colors unless one is in a weakened state. The reversing (opposite) color(s) needs to be utilized for one or more sessions (or at least once a week after a predominant color has been used) to avoid overload of the aura by one color.

If one is using a two-color tonation on various parts of the body, one might get an unfavorable reaction if the two colored lights overlap on the body when simultaneously used. Two colors may be needed, for instance, when an individual suffers from bruises, with one part of the body swollen (requiring the cool spectrum — Indigo) and another part needing a stimulant (the warm spectrum — for example, Red on the liver). When this seems necessary, make sure that the opposite side of the spectrum (warm or cool) is not used during the same tonation but after at least one hour. Simultaneous with the swelling (Indigo), a light fever could be treated by Turquoise (both cool colors). For two-color tonation, see Chapter 4, "Using More Than One Color in a Session."

SEVERING CONNECTION. Obviously there comes a time in life when a person's physical body deteriorates to the point where contemporary medicine or even The 49th Vibrational Technique cannot reverse the destructive or degenerative process. When this time comes, one needs to deal differently with its ramifications, preparing for the person's next state, but even in this case The 49th Vibrational Technique can greatly help ease the transition by reducing pain.

When Cleansing Reactions Are Too Intense

CLEANSING SYMPTOMS. Since an important aspect of The 49th Vibrational Technique is to remove the toxins from the body, a cleansing effort by the eliminative systems will sometimes result. In general one should not be overly concerned, since the system is cooperating intelligently by cleansing itself. In some cases, when one is ridding one's body of toxins, some of the digestive and eliminative functions can be strained.

CONSTIPATION. When constipation occurs, the use of Yellow is generally appropriate for stimulation on the area of the stomach down to the area of the lower intestines (Areas 6, 7, 8, 9, Diagram 5-1).

DIARRHEA. If the opposite (diarrhea) should happen, colors from the blue side of the spectrum should be used to again calm this function. However, Yellow is needed first to rid the body of as many toxins as possible (one session), followed by Turquoise (one session). If diarrhea is still experienced after that, use Indigo on the same areas in repeated sessions until digestion is normalized.

OTHER SYMPTOMS. Minor skin rashes or discomfort in the head area may surface; however, the system is only cleansing itself. If the discomfort becomes excessive, then the tonation should be temporarily halted or an alternative balancing color used. This is why The 49th Vibrational Technique on every seventh tonation of one color or of predominantly warm or cool colors uses an opposite color once. This practice eliminates much of the discomfort that comes from the natural, intense cleansing through color therapy.

FEVERS. The above cleansing symptoms are analogous to the way that fever, for instance, acts in our bodies. When it initially breaks out, it is not necessarily considered a harmful sign, as the fever is basically counteracting much of the oncoming disease. Our first reaction might be to look for help in a bottle of aspirin, but this is not a logical approach unless the fever reaches the 103- to 104-degree range. The same cleansing process found in fevers may happen with color medicine, as the system rids itself of the cause of disease through the vibrational healing process.

THE BODY'S RESPONSE. Generally speaking, the normal body will be able to adequately accept well-programmed color medicine. The nature of the human aura is such that even if color medicine is applied more frequently than necessary, there is generally no harm. That is, a relatively healthy body will not overreact to excessive or even inappropriate colors, since the aura repels unneeded colors. On the other hand, the aura of someone who is very sick might not have the same selectivity as would a healthy one, and a reaction might occur from the use of an inappropriate color if not monitored. In this case, care has to be taken to choose the most effective color(s) for relief.

SEVERE CASES. When one is using color therapy on severe chronic or very acute cases, professional monitoring may be necessary for the number of tonations, the various colors applied, and their appropriate sequence.

In some instances, the detection of weak areas in the body or of hidden causes can be extremely important in terms of determining which systems of the body need color medicine. This vast subject of locating energy blockages in the body is to be covered in a separate manual.

Summary of Body-Area Codes

The abbreviated symbols for larger tonation areas with the twelve colors utilized by The 49th Vibrational Technique, cross-referenced to Diagram 5-1, are:

SF: Systemic Front (from hip joints to above the head on bare skin)

SB: Systemic Back (from hip joints to above the head on bare skin)

AA: Affected Areas (areas showing symptoms on bare skin of these areas only)

WBF: Whole-Body Front (from head to toe on bare skin)

WBB: Whole-Body Back (from head to toe on bare skin)

Remember: Keep the room darkish and the body warm for all tonations. The correct frequencies of the colors are essential.

APPENDIX

The Color Medicine Schedules for
123 Specific Human Disorders

Numbers indicate specific areas (see Diagram 5-1). Medical examination may be needed first.

1. ADENOIDS:
Lemon on SF; Indigo on 1.

2. ALCOHOLISM:
Blue and Magenta on SF; Scarlet on SF and SB if blood circulation is weak.

3. ALLERGIES (Acute):
Lemon on WBF and WBB and Yellow on SF for 2 weeks. Then Orange on SF (instead of Yellow) for 2 weeks. Treat obvious symptoms separately as they appear. Repeat schedule until well. Eliminate all toxins from air space.

4. ALTITUDE SICKNESS:
Blue on SF, Orange on 2, 3 and 11.

5. ALZHEIMER'S DISEASE:
Lemon on SF; Magenta on 1, 2, 3 and 12.

6. APPENDICITIS:
Green on SF; Blue and Indigo on 8 and 9.

7. ARTERIES (Hardening of):
Lemon, Purple and Magenta on SF.

8. ARTHRITIS (Rheumatoid, Acute):
Green and Magenta on SF or SB, including AA; Blue or Indigo on AA; Lemon on AA.

9. ASTHMA:
Purple on 1, 2 and 3; Scarlet on 12.

10. BACK DISORDERS:
Lemon on SB, Indigo on AA.

11. BALDNESS:
Orange on AA; Lemon on SF; Magenta on 1, 2, 3.

12. BLADDER INFECTION:
Green on SF; Indigo on 9 or 13.

13. BLEEDING (Hemorrhaging):
Indigo on AA until bleeding stops. Wound may have to be stitched by a physician. Then Turquoise on SF including AA; Green and Magenta on AA.

14. BLOOD CLOTS:
Lemon and Magenta SF, including AA.

15. BLOOD IN URINE:
Green on SF; Indigo on 9.

16. BLOOD PRESSURE (High):
Lemon and Purple on SF and SB or WBF and WBB; Magenta on 3 and 12.

17. BLOOD PRESSURE (Low):
Lemon and Scarlet on SF and SB or WBF and WBB.

18. BOILS (Furuncles, Carbuncles):
Lemon on SF, including AA and Orange on AA until pus appears and throbbing is felt. Then Green on AA until pus subsides still alternating with Lemon on SF. Then only Turquoise on SF and Indigo on AA.

19. BONE FRACTURES:
Orange and Lemon as close to the fracture as possible (through cast, if necessary) after adjustment.

20. BRONCHITIS (Acute):
Turquoise on SF; Violet on 1, 2, 3.

21. BRUISES:
Indigo on AA for swelling and pain; after relief, Orange and Lemon on AA.

22. BURNS (Heat):
Blue and Indigo on AA, Turquoise on SF, including AA; then Green on AA.

23. BURNS (from Ultraviolet Rays or X-Rays):
With little or no fever, Green on SF, including AA; Red on AA; Turquoise on injured skin. With higher fevers, Blue or Indigo on SF, including AA; Red on AA.

24. CANCER:
Lemon SF, including AA; Indigo on AA.

25. CANKER SORES:
Green on SF and in mouth. With fever, Blue on 1 and in mouth or SF.

26. CATARACTS (Beginning):
Lemon on SF; Lemon and Yellow on 1 for 2 weeks; then Lemon and Orange on 1 for 4 weeks; then Lemon and Red on 1 for 6 weeks. Magenta on 1, 2, 3.

27. CHICKEN POX:
Green and Blue on SF and rash areas; Indigo on bleeding areas.

28. CHILLS:
Green and Blue on SF; Magenta on 3, 12. With fever, Purple on 3.

29. CHOLERA ASIATICA (Preliminary Stage):
Green on SF; Indigo on 4, 5, 6, 7, 8, 9. As long as danger of collapse persists, Scarlet on SF and SB.

30. CIGARETTE SMOKING:
Green on SF to repair damage; Orange and Lemon on 3 and 11.

31. COLD ONSET (Head):
Scarlet on 1, 2, 3 for one session. Then Green on SF; Blue on 1 and 2.

32. CONCUSSION:
Purple on SF; Indigo on 1.

33. CONSTIPATION:
Lemon on SF; Yellow on 4, 5, 6, 7, 8 alternating with Orange on 4, 5, 6, 7, 8 in stubborn cases.

34. COUGH (with Phlegm):
Lemon on SF and 11. With some fever, Green on SF.

35. CYSTIC FIBROSIS:
Lemon on WBF and on pancreas from back (Area 12).

36. DEAFNESS (Ear):
Lemon on SF; Lemon and Yellow on 1 and 10 or on AA.

37. DIABETES MELLITUS:
Lemon on SF; Yellow on 4, 5, 6, 7, 8 and 9; Magenta on WBF.

38. DIARRHEA:
Yellow on 4, 5, 6, 7, 8 and 9 once; then Turquoise on SF once. If still persistent, Indigo on SF until relieved.

39. DRUG ADDICTION:
Green on SF; Magenta or Scarlet on 3 and 12 if heart rate is low.

40. DIPHTHERIA:
Green and Blue on SF; Magenta on 3, 12; Purple on 3 if fever is high.

41. DYSENTERY:
Green on SF; Yellow on 4, 5, 6, 7, 8 and 9 once or twice. Then Indigo on same areas; Green on SF.

42. EARACHE:
Turquoise on SF; Orange on AA. If not improving, try Violet on AA.

43. EPILEPSY:
Purple on SF; Lemon and Yellow on 1 and 10 for 2 weeks; then Lemon and Orange on 1 and 10 for 4 weeks. Repeat if necessary.

44. FLU:
Green and Blue on SF; Magenta on 3.

45. FOOD POISONING:
Green on SF; Magenta on 3.

46. GALLSTONES:
Lemon on SF; Orange on 5 and 6.

47. GANGRENE:
Lemon and Magenta on SF, including AA.

48. GASTROINTESTINAL DISORDERS:
Yellow on 4, 5, 6, 7, 8 ten times; then Turquoise on SF.

49. GLAUCOMA:
Lemon on SF; Indigo on 1; Magenta on 3 and 12.

50. GONORRHEA and SYPHILIS:
Green and Blue on SF until acute symptoms disappear. Then Lemon on SF.

51. GOUT:
Lemon and Magenta on WBF; Scarlet on 12.

52. GUM DISEASE:
Turquoise on SF; Indigo on 1. If chronic, Lemon on SF.

53. HAIR LOSS:
Orange on AA; Lemon on SF; Magenta on 1, 2, 3. Remove all toxins from the air space.

54. HAY FEVER:
Lemon on SF; Turquoise on 1. If there is lack of oxygen, Blue on 1.

55. HEADACHE (Migraine):
Purple on 1, 2, 3 or Scarlet on 1.

56. HEART RATE (Rapid):
Turquoise and Magenta on SF; Purple on 3 and 12.

57. HEART RATE (Slow):
Lemon and Magenta on SF; Scarlet on 3 and 12. Also try WBF and WBB instead on SF.

58. HEMOPHILIA:
Lemon and Magenta on WBF; Indigo on hemorrhaging areas; Red on 5, 6.

59. HEMORRHOIDS:
Lemon on SB; Indigo on 13.

60. HEPATITIS (Acute):
Green and Blue on SF; Red on 5 and 6.

61. HERNIA:
Lemon on SF; Yellow and Indigo on AA.

62. HICCUPS:
Orange on 4, 5, 6, 7; Indigo on back of neck.

63. HYSTERIA:
Blue and Magenta on SF; Green on 1 or SF; Scarlet on 8, 9.

64. IMMUNE DEFICIENCY (A.I.D.S.):
Red or Lemon on WBF and WBB; Yellow on SF; Violet on 4 (spleen).

65. INDIGESTION:
Orange on 4, 5, 6, 7, 8 and 9.

66. INFLAMMATION:
Green and Blue on SF or SB, including AA; Magenta on 3. With high fever or fast pulse rate, Magenta on 12.

67. INSANITY:
Green on 1 or SF, then Magenta on SF.

68. INSOMNIA:
Violet on 1; Purple on 1, 2, 3.

69. KIDNEY STONES:
Lemon and Magenta on SB.

70. KIDNEYS (Acute Inflammation):
Turquoise on SB; Magenta on SF; Scarlet on 12. With high blood pressure, Magenta on 12 instead of Scarlet.

71. LARYNGITIS:
Turquoise on SF; Violet on 1 and 2.

72. LEUKEMIA:
Red and Lemon on WBF, alternating with Magenta on SF and Indigo on possible hemorrhages.

73. LIVER PROBLEMS (Cirrhosis):
Lemon on SF; Red on 5, 6; Magenta on 3, 4, 5, 6, and 12; Indigo on hemorrhaging areas.

74. LUNG CONGESTION:
Turquoise on SF; Blue on 11; Magenta on 3.

75. MENINGITIS (Acute):
Green and Indigo on SB; Magenta on 3. With high fever, Purple on 3.

76. MENSTRUAL CRAMPS:
Orange on 8 and 9; Scarlet on 12.

77. MENSTRUATION (Excessive Flow):
Indigo on 8, 9.

78. MENSTRUATION (Lack of):
Lemon on SF; Green on 1; Scarlet on 8, 9; Magenta on 12.

79. MISCARRIAGE (Potential, Spotting from Miscarriage):
Green on SF; Indigo on 8, 9.

80. MONONUCLEOSIS (Infection):
Green and Blue on SF; Magenta on 3, 12; Yellow on affected lymph areas. When fever is high, Purple on 3.

81. MUMPS:
Green and Blue on SF; later for convalescence Lemon, then Yellow, then Turquoise, all on SF.

82. MUSCULAR CRAMPS:
Orange on AA.

83. NERVOUS SYSTEM (Sensory):
Lemon and Yellow on SF and SB for 2 weeks; then Lemon and Orange on SF and SB for 4 weeks. Repeat if necessary.

84. NOSEBLEEDS:
Indigo on Area 1. Remove toxins from air space.

85. OBESITY:
Lemon on SF; Violet on 6 and 8 for excessive hunger.

86. PARKINSON'S DISEASE:
Lemon and Yellow on 1 and 10 for 2 weeks; Lemon and Orange on 1 and 10 for 4 weeks. Repeat if necessary.

87. PLEURISY:
Green on SF; Blue on 3, 11; Magenta on 3, 12.

88. PNEUMONIA:
Green on SF; Blue on 3 and 11; Magenta on 3. When fever is high, Purple on 3.

89. POLIO:
Green on SF, including AA. With fever, Blue on SF. Also, SF and SB, including AA; Lemon and Yellow for 2 weeks; then Lemon and Orange for 4 weeks; then Lemon and Red for 6 weeks. Repeat if necessary. With muscle problems and weakness, Scarlet on SF, including AA.

90. PREGNANCY (Assumed Normal):
Green on SF; Yellow on 4, 5, 6, 7 and 8; Magenta on 3 and 12.

91. PREGNANCY (Prolonged Labor):
Green on 1; Scarlet on 8, 9.

92. PROSTATE INFLAMMATION (Acute):
Turquoise on SF; Blue between 9 and 13.

93. RABIES:
Stage 1 – Green on SF and SB; Blue on SF; Yellow on SB.
Stage 2 (Excitement) – Yellow on SB only; Magenta on 1-3; Violet on SF.
Stage 3 (Paralytic) – Scarlet on SF and SB.

94. RHEUMATIC FEVERS (Acute):
Green and Indigo on SF, including AA; Magenta on 3, 12.

95. SKIN DISORDERS:
Moist kinds: Turquoise on SF and AA. When drying, Indigo on AA, Turquoise on SF. Dry kinds: Lemon on SF, Orange on AA. When AA becomes moist: tonate as given for moist kinds.

96. SCARLET FEVER:
Green and Blue on SF or SB, including rash areas, Magenta on 3. With high fevers, Purple on 3.

97. SENSORY ABILITY (Loss of):
Lemon on SF or SB; Lemon and Yellow on SF or SB for 2 weeks; Lemon and Orange on SF or SB for 4 weeks; Lemon and Red on SF or SB for 6 weeks. Repeat if necessary.

98. SEXUAL IMPOTENCE:
Green and Orange on SF; Magenta on SF and 12; Scarlet on 8 and 9.

99. SEXUAL OVERACTIVITY:
Turquoise on SF; Purple on 8, 9 and 12; Magenta on SF.

100. SHINGLES:
Acute – Green and Indigo on SB and all AA. Chronic – SB and all AA; Lemon and Yellow for 2 weeks; then Lemon and Orange for 4 weeks. Violet on pain areas. Repeat if necessary.

101. SICKLE-CELL ANEMIA:
Red and Lemon on WBF; Magenta on 3 and 12; Violet on 4.

102. SIGHT PROBLEMS:
Lemon on SF; Yellow on 1 for 2 weeks; then Lemon on SF and Orange on 1 for 4 weeks; then Lemon on SF and Red on 1 for 6 weeks. Repeat if necessary.

103. SINUS INFLAMMATION (Acute):
Green on SF; Blue on 1.

104. SLEEPING SICKNESS:
Yellow and Green on SF and on back of neck; Blue on SF.

105. SPINAL GROWTH:
Indigo on AA alternating with Yellow and Lemon on SB for 2 weeks; then with Lemon and Orange on SB for 4 weeks; then Lemon and Red on SB for 6 weeks. Repeat if necessary.

106. SPLEEN (Activation):
Violet on 4.

107. SPRAINS:
Indigo on AA for pains; then Green on SF and AA; then Orange on AA and a few more sessions of Indigo on AA.

108. STRESS:
Violet on 1; or Purple on 1, 2, 3, if pulse rate is high.

109. STROKE (Paralysis):
Purple on 1, 2, 3 and Indigo on WBF and 10; later Lemon on SF; Magenta on 1, 2, 3.

110. SUNSTROKE/SUNBURN:
Blue on SF; Purple on 3 for sunstroke; however, Red on AA for sunburn.

111. THROAT (Sore, Acute):
Green on SF; Blue on 1 and 2. With high fever, Blue on SF. With headache and high fever, Purple on 1, 2, 3.

112. THYMUS GLAND (Hypertrophy):
Lemon on SF; Indigo on 3 (Thymus).

113. THYROID (Overactivity):
Lemon and Indigo on SF; Green on 1; Purple on 3. With high blood pressure, Purple on SF.

114. THYROID (Underactivity):
Orange and Lemon on SF; Green on 1.

115. TONSILLITIS (Acute):
Green on SF. With high fever, Purple on 1, 2 and 3.

116. TOOTHACHE:
Indigo on 1.

117. *TUBERCULOSIS:*

Lemon and Orange on SF; Orange on 11; Indigo on open areas. With pulmonary hemorrhaging, Purple on 3. With fever, use Turquoise or Green and Blue on SF instead of Lemon and Orange. With high fevers, use Purple on 3. Orange is not used for lymphatic tuberculosis.

118. *TUMORS:*

Lemon on SF, including AA; Indigo on AA; when shrunk and hard, Orange on AA.

119. *THYROID FEVERS:*

Green and Blue on SF; Magenta on 3. With high fevers or headache, Purple on 3.

120. *ULCERS:*

Lemon on SF; Indigo on 4 and 6.

121. *URINE SUPPRESSION:*

Green on SB; Scarlet on 12.

122. *VARICOSE VEINS:*

Lemon and Magenta on SF or SB, including AA; Indigo on AA. Also try Scarlet on AA.

123. *VOMITING:*

Orange on 4, 5, 6. Repeat until only water is vomited; then Indigo on 4, 5, 6.

Quick-reference Checklist For Color Tonation

1. Preheat room to 80° F (28° C) or use electric space heater to warm the body. Set up light and tape player for relaxing music or color/sound vibrational tape.

2. Darken room as much as possible.

3. Prepare area for person to lie on, head pointing toward magnetic north (pole star). (When sitting, back of head is pointing north.)

4. Prepare a clear glass of purified water to be tonated.

5. Choose tonation area of body by symptom and select the appropriate color from schedule (see Appendix).

6. Insert color filter in filter holder at light source, turn on light.

7. Tonation to be applied to bare skin for treatment.

8. Insert appropriate sound tape or healing tape for reinforcement.

9. Quiet the environment and set clock for one-hour tonation.

10. Tonate, relax and enjoy. If there is a feeling of uneasiness, choose a different color, switch to the opposite color or end tonation.

11. Turn off light source promptly after one hour (except for Green or Turquoise, if needed). Continue to relax in darkened room for 5-10 minutes to fully absorb the color vibration.

12. Consume the color-treated water slowly.

13. Do not eat or bathe one hour before or after tonation.

14. Except for emergencies, wait at least 1-3 hours before the next tonation.

Suggested Reading

On Dinshah research:
Dinshah, Ghadiali. *Spectro-Chrome-Metry Encyclopaedia, Vols. 1–3,* Spectro-Chrome Institute, New Jersey, 1939.

On Dinshah color schedules:
Dinshah, Darius. *Let there Be Light,* Dinshah Health Institute, New Jersey, 1985.

On Goethe's theory of color and on water prisms:
Proskauer, Heinrich. *The Rediscovery of Color,* Anthroposophic Press, Spring Valley, New Jersey, 1986.

On chakras:
Leadbeater, C.W. *The Chakras,* The Theosophical Publishing House, Illinois, 1977.

On the aura:
Leadbeater, W.E. *Man Visible and Invisible,* The Theosophical Publishing House, Illinois, 1971.

On etheric body health aura:
Powell, A.E. *The Etheric Double,* The Theosophical Publishing House, Illinois, 1979.

On modern physics:
Talbot, Michael. *Mysticism and the New Physics,* Bantam Books, New York, 1980.

Contact address

Charles Klotsche
c/o The 49th Vibration, Inc., P.O. Box 371, Sedona, AZ 86336, U.S.A.

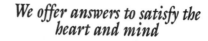

Light Technology Publishing Presents

THE EXPLORER RACE SERIES

The Origin... The Purpose... The Future of Humanity...

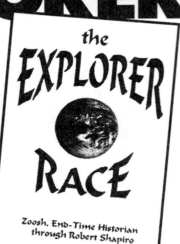

the **EXPLORER** **RACE**

Zoosh, End-Time Historian
through Robert Shapiro

Zoosh & Others through Robert Shapiro

"After all the words that we put out, ultimately the intention is to persuade people's minds, otherwise known as giving their minds the answers that their minds hunger for so that their minds can get out of the way and let their hearts take them to where they would naturally go anyway." – Zoosh/Robert Shapiro

THE SERIES

Humans — creators in training — have a purpose and destiny so heart-warmingly, profoundly glorious that it is almost unbelievable from our present dimensional perspective. Humans are great lightbeings from beyond this creation, gaining experience in dense physicality. This truth about the great human genetic experiment of the Explorer Race and the mechanics of creation is being revealed for the first time by Zoosh and his friends through superchannel Robert Shapiro. These books read like adventure stories as we follow the clues from this creation that we live in out to the Council of Creators and beyond.

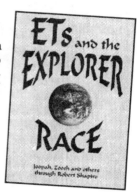
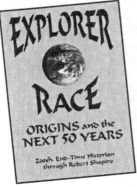

THE EXPLORER RACE SERIES

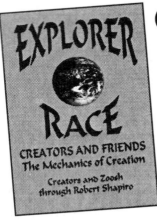

EXPLORER RACE
CREATORS AND FRIENDS
The Mechanics of Creation

Creators and Zoosh
through Robert Shapiro

❹ EXPLORER RACE: Creators and Friends — the Mechanics of Creation

As we explore the greater reality beyond our planet, our galaxy, our dimension, our creation, we meet prototypes, designers, shapemakers, creators, creators of creators and friends of our Creator, who explain their roles in this creation and their experiences before and beyond this creation. As our awareness expands about the way creation works, our awareness of who we are expands and we realize that a part of ourselves is in that vast creation — and that we are much greater and more magnificent than even science fiction had led us to believe. Join us in the adventure of discovery. It's mind-stretching!

435p $19.95

❺ EXPLORER RACE: Particle Personalities

All around you in every moment you are surrounded by the most magical and mystical beings. They are too small for you to see as single individuals, but in groups you know them as the physical matter of your daily life. Particles who might be considered either atoms or portions of atoms consciously view the vast spectrum of reality, yet also have a sense of personal memory like your own linear memory. These particles remember where they have been and what they have done in their infinitely long lives. Some of the particles we hear from are Gold, Mountain Lion, Liquid Light, Uranium, the Great Pyramid's Capstone, This Orb's Boundary, Ice and Ninth-Dimensional Fire.   237p $14.95

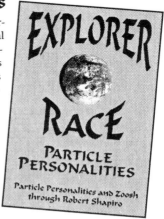

EXPLORER RACE
PARTICLE PERSONALITIES

Particle Personalities and Zoosh
through Robert Shapiro

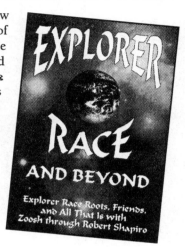

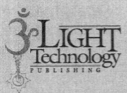
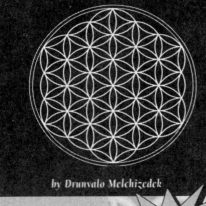

THE
ANCIENT SECRET
OF THE
FLOWER
OF LIFE
VOLUME 2

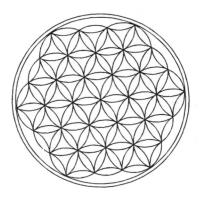

THE
ANCIENT SECRET
OF THE
FLOWER OF LIFE

VOLUME II   *Drunvalo Melchizedek*

COMING SPRING 2000

Here, Drunvalo Melchizedek presents in text and graphics the second half of the Flower of Life Workshop, illuminating the mysteries of how we came to be, why the world is the way it is and the subtle energies that allow our awareness to blossom into its true beauty.

It also explores in great detail the Mer-Ka-Ba, the 55-foot-diameter energy field of the human lightbody. This knowledge leads to ascension and the next dimensional world.

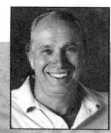

Drunvalo Melchizedek

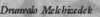

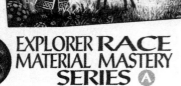

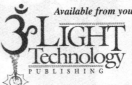

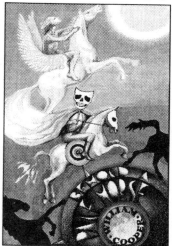
Table of Contents

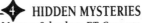
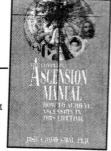

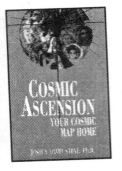

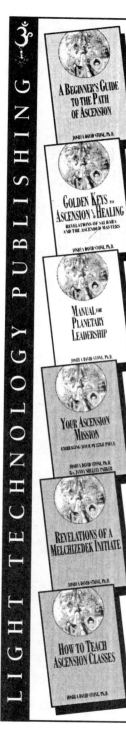

 A BEGINNER'S GUIDE
TO THE PATH OF ASCENSION

This volume covers the basics of ascension clearly and completely, from the spiritual hierarchy to the angels and star beings, in Dr. Stone's easy-to-read style. From his background in psychology he offers a unique perspective on such issues as karma, the transcendence of the negative ego, the power of the spoken word and the psychology of ascension.

$14.95   Softcover 166p   ISBN 1-891824-02-3

 GOLDEN KEYS TO ASCENSION AND HEALING
REVELATIONS OF SAI BABA
AND THE ASCENDED MASTERS

This book represents the wisdom of the ascended masters condensed into concise keys that serve as a spiritual guide. These 420 golden keys present the multitude of methods, techniques, affirmations, prayers and insights Dr. Stone has gleaned from his own background in psychology and life conditions and his thorough research of all the ancient and contemporary classics that speak of the path to God realization.

$14.95   Softcover 206p   ISBN 1-891824-03-1

 MANUAL FOR PLANETARY LEADERSHIP

Here at last is an indispensible book that has been urgently needed in these uncertain times. This book lays out, in an orderly and clear fashion the guidelines for leadership in the world and in one's own life. It serves as a reference manual for moral and spiritual living and offers a vision of a world where strong love and the highest aspirations of humanity triumph.

$14.95   Softcover 284p   ISBN 1-891824-05-8

 YOUR ASCENSION MISSION
EMBRACING YOUR PUZZLE PIECE

This book shows how each person's puzzle piece is just as vital and necessary as any other. Fourteen chapters explain in detail all aspects of living the fullest expression of your unique individuality.

$14.95   Softcover 248p   ISBN 1-891824-09-0

 REVELATIONS OF A MELCHIZEDEK INITIATE

Dr. Stone's spiritual autobiography, beginning with his ascension initiation and progression into the 12th initiation, is filled with insight, tools and information. It will lift you into wondrous planetary and cosmic realms.

$14.95   Softcover   ISBN 1-891824-10-4

 HOW TO TEACH ASCENSION CLASSES

This book serves as an ideal foundation for teaching ascension classes and presenting workshops. The inner-plane ascended masters have guided Dr. Stone to write this book, using his Easy-to-Read-Encyclopedia of the Spiritual Path as a foundation. It covers an entire one- to two-year program of classes.

$14.95 Softcover 136p   ISBN 1-891824-15-5

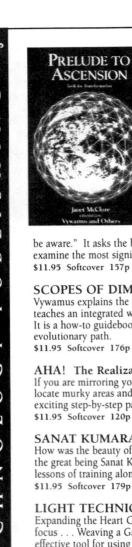

VYWAMUS
JANET MCCLURE

TOOLS FOR TRANSFORMATION

PRELUDE TO ASCENSION
Tools for Transformation
Janet McClure channeling Djwhal Khul, Vywamus & others
Your four bodies, the Tibetan Lesson series, the Twelve
Rays, the Cosmic Walk-in and others. All previously
unpublished channelings by Janet McClure.
$29.95 Softcover 850p . . . . .ISBN 0-929385-54-3

THE SOURCE ADVENTURE
Life is discovery, and this book is a journey of discovery
"to learn, to grow, to recognize the opportunities — to
be aware." It asks the big question, "Why are you here?" and leads the reader to
examine the most significant questions of a lifetime.
$11.95 Softcover 157p . . . . .ISBN 0-929385-06-3

SCOPES OF DIMENSIONS
Vywamus explains the process of exploring and experiencing the dimensions. He
teaches an integrated way to utilize the combined strengths of each dimension.
It is a how-to guidebook for living in the multidimensional reality that is our true
evolutionary path.
$11.95 Softcover 176p . . . . .ISBN 0-929385-09-8

AHA! The Realization Book (with Lilian Harben)
If you are mirroring your life in a way that is not desirable, this book can help you
locate murky areas and make them "suddenly . . . crystal clear." Readers will find it an
exciting step-by-step path to changing and evolving their lives.
$11.95 Softcover 120p . . . . .ISBN 0-929385-14-4

SANAT KUMARA Training a Planetary Logos
How was the beauty of this world created? The answer is in the story of Earth's Logos,
the great being Sanat Kumara. A journey through his eyes as he learns the real-life
lessons of training along the path of mastery.
$11.95 Softcover 179p . . . . .ISBN 0-929385-17-9

LIGHT TECHNIQUES That Trigger Transformation
Expanding the Heart Center . . . Launching your Light . . . Releasing the destructive
focus . . . Weaving a Garment of Light . . . Light Alignment & more. A wonderfully
effective tool for using light to transcend. Beautiful guidance!
$11.95 Softcover 145p . . . . .ISBN 0-929385-00-4

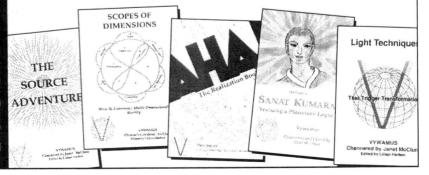

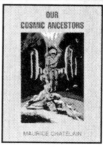
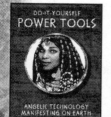
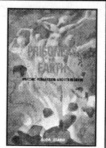
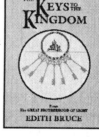
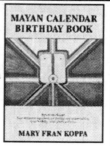

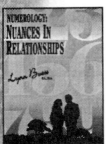
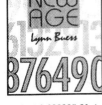
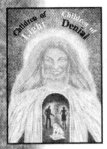
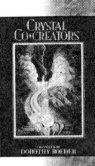
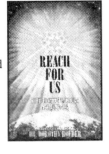

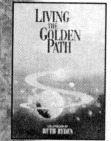
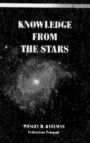

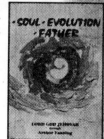
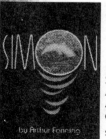

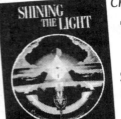
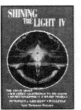
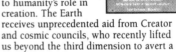
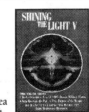

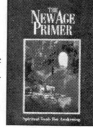
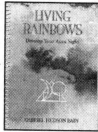
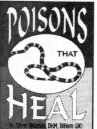
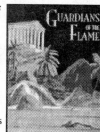
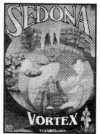

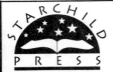
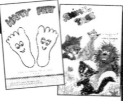
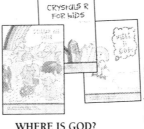
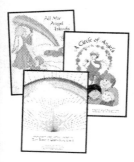
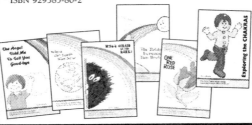

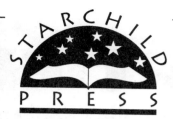

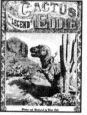
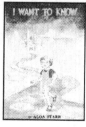
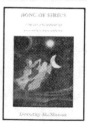

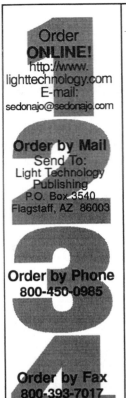
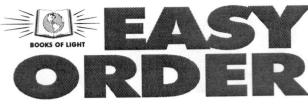

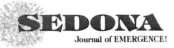

Notes

Notes

Notes

Notes

Notes

Notes

Notes

Notes

Notes

Notes